2. 00

D1461684

Champion of
Homoeopathy

Champion of Homoeopathy

THE LIFE OF
MARGERY BLACKIE

Constance Babington Smith

JOHN MURRAY

© Constance Babington Smith 1986

First published 1986
by John Murray (Publishers) Ltd
50 Albemarle Street, London W1X 4BD

Typeset by Inforum Ltd, Portsmouth
Printed and bound in Great Britain
by The Bath Press, Avon

British Library CIP data
Babington Smith, Constance
Champion of homoeopathy : the life
of Margery Blackie.
1. Blackie, Margery G.   2. Homoeopathic
physicians—Great Britain—Biography
I. Title
615.5'32'0924   RX66.B5
ISBN 0–7195–4263–4

CONTENTS

ILLUSTRATIONS

THANKS AND ACKNOWLEDGEMENTS are given for the use of the
following illustrations: Associated Press Ltd, 17; Lt. Col. M.C.
Barraclough, 16; Blackie Foundation Trust, 1, 6, 10, 11, 13, 21;
Mr Brian Blackie, 3; Haberdashers' Aske's School, 4; Harrison
& Laking Ltd, 20; Homoeopathic Trust for Research and Edu-
cation, 9; The Hon. Thomas Lindsay, 14; Portman Press
Bureau, 15; Rawood Ltd, 18; Royal Free Hospital, 7, 8; Mrs
Ruth Shute, 12; Mrs Mollie Symonds, 5.

AUTHOR'S NOTE

During the writing of this book many of Dr Blackie's patients have given me encouragement and help that I deeply appreciate, and in the first place I express my gratitude to Her Majesty the Queen for her interest, and for her gracious permission to quote extracts from two letters, one of them from herself to Dr Blackie, the other from His Majesty King George VI to Sir John Weir. In addition I am warmly grateful to Her Majesty Queen Elizabeth the Queen Mother for her heartening enthusiasm for my project. Another member of the royal family to whom I am specially indebted is Her Royal Highness Princess Alice, Duchess of Gloucester. She gave generously of her time to talk with me about Dr Blackie, and later she read and approved passages of my draft. Recollections of Dr Blackie as a member of the Royal Medical Household were kindly shared with me by Sir Richard Bayliss, and I am also very grateful to Dr Charles Elliott, Dr Blackie's successor as Physician to Her Majesty the Queen, for his memories as well as for his constant interest in my book.

The idea that a biography of Margery Blackie should be written was suggested to me some years ago by one of her patients, Lady Namier. At the time I was engaged on another book, and I did not actually meet Dr Blackie. But after her death in 1981, when I was free to undertake the work, I got into touch with two of her colleagues, Dr Anita Davies and Dr Ronald Davey. I then contacted members of the Blackie family – Mr Brian Blackie, Mrs Mollie Symons and Mrs Lillian Townend – and with their approval and assistance, for which I am happy to thank them, I was able to embark on the preliminary research.

At this early stage I met the person who more than anyone else has enabled me to collect the information necessary for writing the biography, Mrs Joyce Westmorland. As a close friend to Dr Blackie and Miss Musette Majendie during their final years at Hedingham Castle, she had become responsible for many albums, letters, photographs and other material. Furthermore she was well acquainted with Dr Blackie's family, colleagues and friends, as well as with some of Miss Majendie's relatives. I cannot thank her enough for her help and hospitality. At her home I was able to have long talks with many who had known Dr Blackie. She also took me in her car for interviews as far afield as Kent and Cornwall.

This account of Dr Blackie's life and work could not possibly have been written without extensive briefing from a number of the leading homoeopathic doctors who had worked closely with her. I must emphasise my indebtedness to all of them, especially to Dr Alastair Jack for his wise and kindly advice, for the loan of a major series of Dr Blackie's letters, and for his most helpful criticism of my first complete draft. To Dr Anita Davies I am particularly grateful for her reminiscences, for her advice on the rendering of case histories, and for introducing me to Mrs Janet Bodman, who kindly gave me access to an important series of letters from Dr Blackie to the late Dr Frank Bodman. In addition I would like to thank all of Dr Blackie's other colleagues who gladly spoke to me about her. These included Dr Ronald Davey, Dr Max Deacon, Dr Donald Foubister, Dr John Hughes-Games, Dr Frank Johnson and Dr Kathleen Priestman. Another who must be mentioned here is Mr John Ainsworth, whose advice on homoeopathic pharmacology was uniquely helpful. Several of these experts helped me by suggesting corrections to my drafts. My thanks are also due to those of Dr Blackie's patients and their relatives who were kind enough to describe, by letter or in conversation, their memories of her treatments. Where I have quoted from what they told me I have in most cases withheld their names.

A number of Dr Blackie's friends and acquaintances advised me on various matters connected with her work, and I am sincerely grateful to the following: Lt Col Michael Barraclough, Miss Jo Hiscox, and Miss Mari Price of the Homoeopathic Trust for Research and Education; Miss Lily Bottom of the Missionary School of Medicine; Mr Anthony Dove and Mr Leonard Knowles, formerly of the Royal London Homoeopathic Hospital; Mr Robin Holland-Martin of the Blackie Foundation Trust; Mrs Anne Barraclough, secretary to Dr Blackie. I would also like to mention my warm gratitude to Dr Edith Gilchrist, Archivist of the Royal Free Hospital, Mrs Jill Norman of the Haberdashers' Aske's School, and Mr Peter Crown of Lachasse Ltd, all of whom briefed me in their specialised fields.

For insight into Dr Blackie's personal relationships I acknowledge the help of the Hon Thomas Lindsay, the Hon Vera Grenfell, Miss Dorothy Meynell, and Mrs Dinah Estep (relatives of Miss Majendie); Mrs Ella Hart (sister of Dr Helena Banks) and Mrs Margaret Evans (Dr Banks's niece); Mrs Ruth Shute (daughter of Dr Campbell Morgan); Mrs Bethan Lloyd-Jones (widow of Dr Martyn Lloyd-Jones) and Lady Catherwood (his daughter); also of Mrs Clare Menglides (daughter of Mrs Susanna MacMichael, *née* Bernard).

Throughout my work I relied upon *The British Homoeopathic Journal* for documentary evidence, and I am grateful to the Council of the Faculty of Homoeopathy for permission to quote from the *Journal*, especially from the issues that cover the period of Dr Blackie's professional life. I must also thank the Trustees of the Blackie Foundation Trust for permission to quote from Dr Blackie's book *The Patient, Not the Cure* (now reissued by Unwin Paperbacks as *The Challenge of Homoeopathy*). The paragraph from *The Times* on Margery's royal appointment is quoted with the permission of Times Newspapers Ltd, and permission has been given by the *British*

Medical Journal for the quotation from their review of *The Patient, Not the Cure*. For quotations from letters to Dr Blackie I am glad to acknowledge permissions from the Hon Thomas Lindsay (letter from Lady Jane Lindsay), Dr Frank Johnson, Dr June Burger, Dr Dorothy West, and the Iulia de Beausobre Estate (letters from Lady Namier).

Finally I would like to thank my publisher Mr John Murray for his personal supervision of the book, and for suggesting that a non-homoeopathic doctor should read the typescript. Dr John Horder, formerly President of the Royal College of General Practitioners, kindly agreed to do so, and thanks to his comments I was enabled to avoid several errors, and also to make some needful modifications to the text. I am truly grateful to him.

CONSTANCE BABINGTON SMITH

Cambridge 1985

PART ONE

Learning

Early Years

Homoeopathy was in her blood. As a child Margery Blackie was given homoeopathic remedies as a matter of course, and she herself, looking back long afterwards, declared that she was 'one of those lucky people who absorbed homoeopathy in the nursery'.

But besides this, a close relative of hers had been an untiring upholder of 'the cause'. Her uncle by marriage James Compton Burnett (father of the novelist) had been one of the great fighters for homoeopathy of his day. He was a ferocious campaigner, at a time when there was need for courage. In nineteenth-century Britain, outside the circles of devotees, homoeopaths were despised, ridiculed and slandered, and there was a real danger that their speciality would be suppressed as illegal.

Margery never knew her uncle – a big, bearded man with a vehement temperament – he died in 1901 when she was three. But the influence of his achievements lived on. His innumerable therapeutic successes (often hailed as miracles) in treating illnesses and ailments ranging from catarrh to cancer, from angina to hiccoughs, the permanent importance of his researches, his inspiring enthusiasm as a teacher, his polemics as editor of the *Homoeopathic World*, his prolific writings – all these contributed to the Blackie family's unwavering belief in homoeopathic medicine. And they may well have helped to give rise to a cherished family legend that Margery, at the age of five (or even three, it was sometimes claimed) announced that she intended to be a doctor.

'Uncle James' had espoused homoeopathy after becoming intensely disillusioned with the medical methods of his time. In tune with his passionate nature, he likened his 'conversion' to that of St Paul on the Damascus Road. And he himself put on record how it came about. The following account is taken from the opening pages of a booklet he wrote entitled 'Fifty Reasons for being a Homoeopath'.

One wintry afternoon, in the Glasgow hospital where he was working as a young doctor in the 1870s, he was busy writing out death certificates when a small corpse was carried past the surgery window. He turned to the old dispenser and said, 'Tim, who's that dead now?' 'Little Georgie, Sir,' was the answer. Little Georgie was a waif who belonged to nobody but was beloved by everyone; he had been kept in odd beds as one might keep a pet animal. A few days previously a bed had been wanted for an acute case, and little Georgie had been moved from his warm snug corner to a bed that was in front of a window. There he caught cold. Pleurisy followed and now he was a corpse.

Dr Compton Burnett was shattered. '*I felt sure that he need not have died,*' he wrote, 'and the consciousness nearly pressed me down into the earth . . . If I could only have stopped the initial fever that followed the chill by the window, Georgie had probably lived.' That evening he happened to be seeing a friend who was an enthusiast for homoeopathy and he confessed that he had almost decided to abandon his medical career – he would emigrate to America and take up farming. The friend persuaded him to delay his decision, and to look into homoeopathy with an open mind, although this would, of course, be far from easy for one who had been taught that it was 'therapeutic nihilism'. After many hesitations and with secret feelings of guilt Dr Compton Burnett obtained two books recommended by his friend, and from them he learnt just how radically the whole concept of homoeopathy differed from accepted medical theory. For homoeopathic therapy does not make a direct attack upon the symptoms of a disease

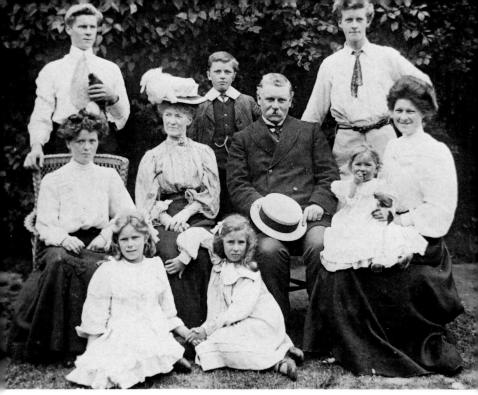

1 Margery (sitting on the
ground, *l*) with her parents
and members of her family

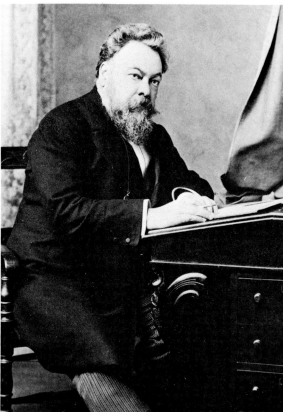

2 Dr James Compton Burnett

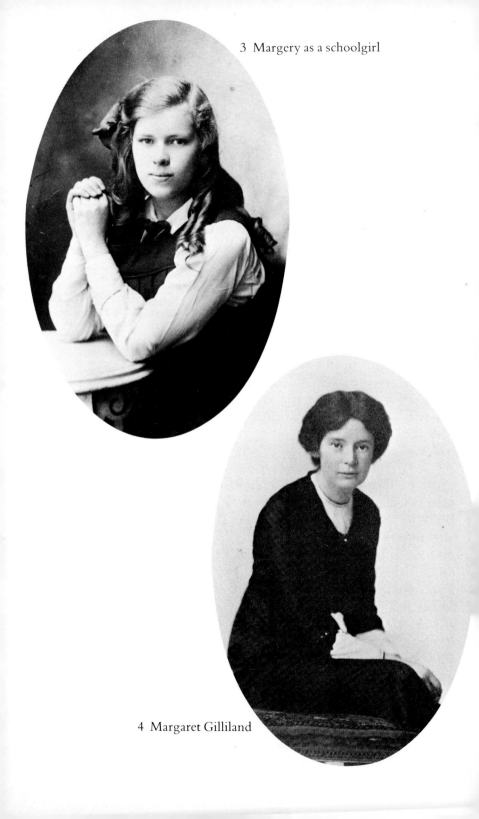

3 Margery as a schoolgirl

4 Margaret Gilliland

by means of antidotes. Instead it stimulates the patient's natural potentialities of resistance to the disease by means of minute amounts of medical substances (many of them, but by no means all, derived from herbal tinctures) which in a healthy person would cause the very same disease. In the words of Margery Blackie herself, written many years later, 'Like should be treated by like . . . This is the basis of homoeopathy.' This fundamental principle is a concept that can be readily understood by comparison with such methods as vaccination or the use of controlled radiation in the treatment of cancer.

After a week or two Dr Compton Burnett had mastered the general idea. But he was unconvinced. 'No,' he said to himself, 'I could not be a homoeopath.' He decided however that he would try out the method at the bedside, prove it to be a lying sham, and expose it to an admiring profession. So he resolved to experiment by administering what might be called homoeopathic first aid. He would test the claim that simple fever could be cut short with *Aconite*.★ 'Ah,' he thought, 'if that is true, *Aconite* would have saved little Georgie.'

At the time he was in charge of a ward where children who had been taken ill, mostly with feverish colds or chills, were put till their diseases had declared themselves (then they were drafted off to other wards). This gave him the chance he needed. He put a few drops of tincture of *Aconite* into a large bottle of water and handed it to the nurse who was looking after the ward, with instructions to give some to all the cases on one side of the ward as soon as they were brought in. Those on the other side were not to have the *Aconite* solution, but were to be treated in the usual way. At his next morning visit, so he claimed, he found that nearly all the children on the *Aconite* side had normal temperatures and were playing about in their beds. Those on the non-*Aconite* side were worse or about the same. 'And so it went on day after day. Those that got *Aconite* were generally convalescent in twenty-four or

★ A homoeopathic remedy prepared from *Aconitum napellus* (monk's hood).

forty-eight hours.' 'For a little while I was simply dumb-
founded,' he wrote, 'and I spent much of my nights studying
homoeopathy; I had no time during the day.'

He had not told the nurse anything about the contents of his
big bottle, which she nicknamed 'Dr Burnett's fever bottle'.
Then one morning, after he had twice had to miss his round,
the nurse seemed rather quiet when he entered the children's
ward, and she told him 'with a certain forced dutifulness' that
all the cases might, she thought, be dismissed. 'Indeed,' he
said, 'how's that?' 'Well, doctor,' she answered, 'as you did
not come round on Sunday or yesterday, I gave your fever
medicine to them all; and indeed I had not the heart to see you
go on with your cruel experiments any longer; you are like all
the young doctors that come here – you are only trying
experiments!' 'Very well, nurse,' replied the doctor, 'give the
medicine in future to all that come in.'

Dr Compton Burnett's niece, Margery Grace Blackie, was the
youngest, much the youngest, of a family of ten (her mother
was forty-five when she was born). Her father Robert Blackie
had Scottish ancestry – he belonged to the same 'clan' as the
well-known Edinburgh professor and man of letters, John
Stuart Blackie – and her mother was Welsh. They were living
in Hertfordshire, in the village of Redbourn, at the time of
Margery's birth on 4 February 1898, but the Blackies had no
permanent roots there; it was one of the many places in the
south of England where they lived for a time. They seldom
remained in the same house for long. Margery's father enjoyed moving, and the impulse to uproot his family and plant
them somewhere new seems to have been a compulsive mania
with him. But the family's frequent moves were also necessi-
tated by the need to economise, since Robert Blackie had no
professional work; in formal documents his occupation is
given as 'none', though he is sometimes described as 'of independent means'. These independent means were constantly
dwindling, for he had no business sense. Unsophisticated

by nature, he was gullible and easily duped, or as it has been more kindly put 'he believed in people'.

At one time there had been plenty of money in the family. Margery's paternal grandfather, Robert Blackie Sr, after migrating from Scotland to Liverpool had built up a prosperous engineering business and had acquired valuable land in the suburbs of the city. Then in 1850, after the death of his first wife, he married a distant cousin, Georgiana Pudney, who owned property in Essex near Great Clacton, which was soon to be developed as a seaside resort. Thus the family's home near Liverpool, Litherland Hall, where Margery's father grew up, was a place of considerable affluence.

Liverpool was then in the heyday of its prosperity as Britain's leading seaport. It was also a stronghold of homoeopathic developments, almost as important a centre as London, and in Liverpool James Compton Burnett first established himself as a successful practitioner in 1874. After the little Georgie incident and its sequel he felt he had no choice but to become a homoeopath, which meant professional suicide as far as a normal career in medicine was concerned. So he left Glasgow and in Liverpool launched out afresh. In Liverpool, too, Margery's father became a convinced believer in homoeopathy, and this brought him into touch with other enthusiasts including Dr Compton Burnett.

In those days homoeopaths and their families held closely together and often intermarried. Thus Robert Blackie, at twenty-two, met his future wife Elizabeth ('Lizzie') Rees, the beautiful young daughter of a Welsh civil engineer and architect (later Mayor of Dover) Rowland Rees, whose family believed ardently in homoeopathy and were also devout Wesleyan Methodists. Lizzie's younger sister Katharine (Margery's 'Aunt Katie'), also a beauty, became Dr Compton Burnett's second wife.

Margery's parents, who were married in 1875, made their first home at Pyrford in Surrey, where they took a fine Queen Anne house, The Grange, and their two eldest children,

Elizabeth and Robert, were born there. But in 1879 they moved to Great Clacton and Robert Blackie plunged into speculation in land – this was one of a number of ill-fated business ventures. The family remained there for fifteen years, moving from house to house and growing steadily in numbers with each new baby. But then they went on to Lewisham, and later to Redbourn.

The Blackies' choice of successive homes, although dictated mainly by the need to economise, was also guided by another consideration: was there a Wesleyan chapel nearby? Margery's father was an energetic lay preacher, a respected figure in one Wesleyan community after another, described by a member of his congregation as 'a good Christian gentleman'. He was well built, a handsome man with a walrus moustache, a breezy manner and a ready smile, and one can well picture him holding forth, intent on saving souls from hell-fire, popery and drink (the Blackies themselves were of course strict tee-totallers).

At this time Robert Blackie was still well-to-do, and he aspired to a political career; in 1905 he joined the National Liberal Club. He had acquaintances among the aristocracy and was in demand for shooting parties. Ivy Compton-Burnett, in two of her books, has given somewhat malicious sketches of her uncle. In her first novel *Dolores* 'Mr Blackwood', who had 'a straitened income and a large family', cultivated the air of a prosperous country squire. His wife thought he looked like a member of parliament, and he himself liked to recall that on several occasions in the train he had been taken for one. As a young man he had in fact imagined that he was destined for a career in politics but 'family losses following his early marriage had cancelled the prospect'. Urged on by his wife, 'whose zeal for religion and temperance did not fall short of her husband's', Mr Blackwood spent most of his time addressing meetings in 'loud and fervid discourse'. But he had another side as well: 'There was much that was gentle and genial about Mr Blackwood. Any labouring man of the district . . . would have told you that he was "a real gentleman".' This last comment tallies exactly with tributes to Margery's father that were collected after his death.

The second portrayal of Robert Blackie by his niece – a slighter sketch – is in her novel *Men and Wives*. There 'Sir Godfrey Haslam', who came of dissenting stock and was used to 'religious officiation' as head of the house, reads aloud from the Bible at family prayers, then falls on his knees to utter extempore petitions for members of the family and household. This was, of course, the normal daily routine in the Blackie home, as in every Methodist home of the period.

Margery's father, like Sir Godfrey, commanded respect in the Victorian manner. But it was her mother, little Lizzie Blackie, who really ruled the family. Animated and decisive, with a neat figure, lovely hair and a very pretty face, she was, like her father the Dover Mayor, a strong personality. Gifted with a quick mind and a good memory, she liked to show off her intellectual prowess; in this her husband was no rival – Robert Blackie had no academic leanings. She was also proud of her ancestry. One of her forebears, her grandfather John Rees, who had left Wales in Napoleon's time and come to Essex as Clerk of the Works to the Royal Engineers, had supervised the building of eleven Martello Towers, intended to withstand the threatened invasion. Furthermore it could be claimed (according to Margery's aunt Mrs Compton Burnett) that in the more distant past the family had royal lineage. Aunt Katie used to say that they were descended from a princely Welshman, Ap Rees ap Rees ap Madoc.

In *Dolores* Margery's mother is caricatured as a cultural snob. 'Mrs Blackwood', a small sharp-featured woman with an energy of manner and movement 'which belied a delicate form', was generally regarded as 'an affable and clever lady'. But although she was 'a woman of some quickness of feeling and intelligence and some lack of depth in both', she had 'a reverence for intellect and a desire to be held intellectual' which caused some embarrassment to her family.

Thus Ivy Compton-Burnett, in her novels, subjected her uncle and aunt to spiteful ridicule. But in real life, viewed objectively, Robert and Elizabeth Blackie were a happily married couple – they lived to celebrate their diamond wedding – a man and wife who were faithful to the tradition of the Wesleyan ethos. In the Blackie home the ideals of Christian service were strongly to the fore. Thus although Margery's parents were increasingly handicapped financially, and often on the move, the setting of her youth was a stable one of enduring love and piety.

An understanding of Margery's noncomformist background is vitally important for an understanding of her own personality. For many of her characteristics – her dependence upon the Bible for daily inspiration, her self-discipline, her dedication to her patients – can be seen to stem from childhood roots.

Among the Blackie family photographs there is a group taken when Margery was about two, and this is our earliest glimpse of her. Perched on her mother's knee she is a plump, rather plain little toddler, with a look of firm determination on her face. This purposeful expression is noticeable in all the early photographs, and it is clear that, although Margery's looks were very different from those of her pretty mother, she had inherited her mother's masterful character.

As a girl Margery's likeness in looks to her father became evident – she had the same broad face, large features and full lips – but she had her mother's soft wavy hair, sometimes curled into ringlets falling on to her shoulders, sometimes brushed gently back. Though she was certainly not beautiful she was a good-looking young girl, with an engaging directness of demeanour.

She was so much younger than her brothers and sisters that there were no close companionships for her within the family. But she was specially fond of two of her brothers, the youngest, Alan (who teased her), and 'Bob', the eldest. Bob was a charmer with winning manners, even to his little sister. But since he was twenty years her senior he seemed to belong to a different generation. This was also true of her four sisters; the eldest, Elizabeth ('Liz'), had married at twenty-three in the year after Margery's birth.

How providential for Margery that Liz soon had a child – a daughter – for it meant that she and her niece, Mollie Nott, who were very nearly the same age, were able to become playmates and friends. A photograph of the two taken at Wallington near Croydon, where the Blackies were living when Margery was about seven – after an interim at Harpenden – shows them posed together like affectionate little sisters.

After Wallington the Blackies moved to Southend, and when Margery was twelve, in 1910, she was a pupil at the now defunct Alexandra College at Westcliff on Sea. It is interesting that the daughter of the Salvation Army's General Booth, Mrs Booth-Clibborn, renowned as an evangelical preacher ('the Marechale'), was living in Westcliff at this time, and she and her family were good friends of the Blackies. Another family friend, who is said to have influenced Margery and encouraged her ambition to be a doctor, was a medical missionary from China named Cooper.

In 1911 the Blackies made a move which was a landmark in Margery's life. They migrated to West London, and this enabled her to become a day girl at the Haberdashers' Aske's School in Acton, a recently built establishment belonging to an ancient charitable foundation.* (Acton had once been a busy little village on the London–Oxford road, but years before the Blackies arrived it had been developed as an industrial

---

* There was a long history behind the school. In 1688 the Worshipful Company of Haberdashers, a Livery Guild of the City of London, received a bequest from one of its members, Robert Aske, for the purpose of establishing an almshouse and a school for boys. These were originally in Hoxton, but at the end of the nineteenth century new schools were built, one for boys in Hampstead, the other for girls in Acton. At the present time both schools are at Elstree, where the charity purchased the Aldenham House Estate in 1959.

suburb.) She was there for the next six years, so between the ages of thirteen and eighteen, although the family continued moving house – they had three successive addresses in Acton – her school attendance gave a steady continuity to her life. Those six years also meant that the formative time of her adolescence was spent entirely in urban surroundings, thus she naturally grew up with the outlook, the habits, and the interests of a town-dweller, not a country girl. And she was a happy town-dweller, popular at school and 'a jolly girl' – this is how one of her contemporaries remembers her.

The school, belonging as it did to a charity, cultivated high moral standards, and its motto was that of the Worshipful Company of Haberdashers, 'Serve and Obey'. But since it was non-denominational there was no chapel, and on special occasions the girls, who in Margery's day numbered five hundred, ranging from tiny tots to the big girls in the upper school, used to troop off in crocodiles to the nearby Anglican church or to the Wesleyan chapel.

At the time when Margery was there the school was dominated by an outstanding headmistress, Miss Margaret Gilliland. Much admired by the teenage Margery, she was a charming, youthful-looking woman of great integrity. But, for all her charm, she could be fierce with transgressors, and discipline in the school was very strict. One of the rules was that not a word might be spoken in the passages or cloakrooms, and the girls always had to behave 'with the utmost decorum'. Yet Miss Gilliland was by no means an unfeeling martinet. Although she insisted on a high standard of scholarship she strongly believed that her girls must not be put under pressure. She wanted them to become 'intelligent, good-mannered young women, potential home-makers with lively interests outside the limits of the school syllabus'.

She prided herself on knowing each one of her girls and on being aware of their individual abilities, so she doubtless knew that Margery was musical; in the school orchestra she was one of the first violins. Margery was also a keen member of the

Nature Study Society, and the headmistress, who was the society's president, may well have heard her when she gave what was, so far as we know, the first public speech of her life. At a meeting of the Nature Study Society on 24 March 1914, so it was reported in the school magazine, Margery Blackie read 'a very clear and instructive paper' on birds and their eggs.

In this context it is of interest that the Society had been allocated some plots in the school garden for outside experiments, and during that same spring term four of the plots were divided into strips and a different kind of manure or soil was dug into each. Then similar vegetable and flower seeds were sown in each strip, and it was hoped by these experiments to discover which soils were best suited to the various plants. At the last meeting of the term – Margery was by this time one of the two captains in the Upper Fourth Form – there was a 'naming competition' in which members were asked to name leaves, flowers and plants. She probably did well in this competition for she had a remarkably good memory. In later life it was frequently commented upon, and she attributed it to the training she had had as a little girl from her mother, who used to send her shopping without a shopping list. 'The way to a lazy memory is to write things down,' Lizzie Blackie used to say. 'You have to *train* yourself to remember.'

Margery was sixteen and a half when war was declared. For her parents, with four sons of military age, the shock can well be imagined. For Margery herself the routine of home and school continued much as usual: she was now about to enter the 'matriculation form', to prepare for the crucial examination that she had to pass if she was really going to train to be a doctor. So she had months of concentrated hard work ahead. But since it was wartime, and the school had been recognised by the War Office as a voluntary organisation, she and all the girls were kept busy contributing to the war effort, knitting and making garments for servicemen and refugees. It is on record that, at one point, the school sent off 2,243 pairs of mittens, 813 mufflers, and 919 pairs of socks.

In the matriculation form Margery became great friends with one of her classmates, Grace Pollard, and Miss Pollard has some interesting memories. She confirms that Margery always wanted to be a doctor, though she does not recall any mention of homoeopathy. She also remembers that she was extremely proud of having Scottish blood, and insisted that her name must be spelt in the Scottish way; 'Marjorie' was an inferior English spelling. And when she was once asked what she would like for her birthday she said she would much like a copy of *Anne of Geierstein* to complete her collection of Walter Scott novels.

The main event which the war brought for Margery was a joyful one. Her niece Mollie, by now fourteen, had been a day girl at a school in Eastbourne. But on the outbreak of war it had been decided that she should come to Acton to stay with her Blackie grandparents, and should join Margery at the Haberdashers' School. She was of course in a lower form, but at home the two girls were constantly together and their companionship was a happiness for both of them. Temperamentally the two were very different. According to Mollie (now Mrs Symons) Margery was 'always a worker' who took her studies seriously, while she, on the other hand, was much more easygoing.

So Margery was always a worker! But what of her academic record? It was average though not above average. In 1916 she was one of the sixteen girls at her school who passed the matriculation examination of London University, but she was not one of the five who obtained honours certificates, nor did she gain any distinctions. What matter? The one thing which did matter was that the door was now open to her to become a medical student.

Medical Student

Margery's ambition to be a doctor had been warmly encouraged by her parents, and since enthusiasm for homoeopathy was so strong in the family it was taken for granted that she would follow in the footsteps of her famous uncle, and aim at practising one day as a homoeopath.

Even as a girl she must have been familiar with the homoeopathic background. Doubtless she knew that, although the principle of like curing like was as old as Hippocrates, the 'father of modern homoeopathy' was the eighteenth-century German doctor and chemist Samuel Hahnemann, a man of genius who had been so dissatisfied with the medicine of his day that when he stumbled upon the homoeopathic principle he resolved to devote his life to pursuing and applying it. Margery herself, after a lifetime as a homoeopath, summed up Hahnemann's achievement in a telling phrase: 'It has often been said that homoeopathy existed before Hahnemann. So it did; in the same way that gravity existed before Newton.'

The natural law that like cures like had been the first of the great discoveries made by Hahnemann, or more precisely it was a *rediscovery*, for throughout the history of medicine the use of homoeopathic therapeutics has perennially recurred. The story of his discovery has been told many times, but it deserves retelling, for it illustrates in a striking way the whole basis of the homoeopathic method. Hahnemann was not only a physician and chemist but an accomplished linguist and, while translating an English work into German, he found himself questioning the author's assertions as to the action of quinine (*Cinchona*), which in small amounts had already been found very successful in the treatment of malaria – 'intermittent fever' as it was then called. He decided to experiment on himself (he was in good health, and not in the least feverish) by taking large doses of the tincture. For several days he took these doses daily. 'My feet and fingertips etc. at first became cold'. He afterwards wrote.

> I became languid and drowsy; then my heart began to palpitate; my pulse became hard and quick; and intolerable anxiety and trembling (but without a rigor); prostration in all the limbs; then pulsation in the head, redness of the cheeks, thirst; briefly all the symptoms usually associated with intermittent fever appeared in succession, yet without the actual rigor. To sum up: all those symptoms which to me are typical of intermittent fever, as the stupefaction of the senses, a kind of rigidity of all joints, but above all the numb, disagreeable sensation which seems to have its seat in the periosteum [membrane which envelops the bones] over all the bones of the body – all made their appearance. This paroxysm lasted from two to three hours every time, and recurred when I repeated the dose and not otherwise. I discontinued the medicine and I was once more in good health.

So here was proof of a natural law! He had discovered that quinine, an effective remedy for intermittent fever if taken in very small quantities, produced symptoms akin to those of this same fever when taken in larger amounts by a healthy person. He went on to carry out many more such 'provings', experimenting on himself, his family and friends, testing the effects of many different substances upon persons in good health. And thereafter his findings enabled him to conduct further experiments demonstrating that minuscule quantities of these same substances had a therapeutic action. Thus were laid the foundations of the homoeopathy that Margery was to learn and practise. After Hahnemann, his disciples and their successors continued exploring the therapeutic potential of natural substances, building on the foundations that Hahnemann himself had laid. Today more than two thousand medicines are listed in the homoeopathic *materia medica*, the compendium of remedies (according to toxicology, proving studies and clinical experience) which is the homoeopath's vade mecum.

For Margery there was no short cut to becoming a qualified homoeopathic practitioner. As a first step she would have to train in general medicine, and in the summer of 1917 the initial move was made when she applied for admission to the London (Royal Free Hospital) School of Medicine for Women, one of the medical schools belonging to London University.* There was good reason for her choice; at this time no other medical school in London accepted women for complete courses of training, that is, for five-and-a-half year courses which included three years of clinical studies.† True she could have opted for a school in Scotland or in the provinces, but London was obviously preferable for family reasons.

Prejudice against women in the medical profession was still very strong, although nearly half a century had passed since the first great battles for the recognition of women as doctors in Britain had been fought and won: the School of Medicine for Women had been founded in 1874 by one of the most forceful of the pioneers, Sophia Jex-Blake. In the beginning the students had had no access to clinical instruction, but very soon the nearby Royal Free Hospital had agreed to admit women students to its wards, and thus began the long and fruitful association between the hospital and the school. In Margery's time they were located conveniently close to one another in Bloomsbury, the hospital in Gray's Inn Road, in premises that had formerly been a barracks, and the school in Hunter Street.‡

Margery was nineteen when she embarked eagerly on her

* At that time the school accepted women only; it became coeducational in 1948 at the inauguration of the NHS.
† After the war began, however, a few London hospitals allowed women to enter their wards for specialised clinical experience.
‡ Both hospital and school are now in Hampstead.

university course as a medical student. It was a joyful time for her; one of her contemporaries can still remember 'her pleasant fair face and happy expression'. With her hair up in a bun, and skirts to her ankles, she commuted at first from Acton. But after her first year she had a longer journey each day, for she was still living at home and her parents had moved to Redhill.

The Blackies had simultaneously taken an upward leap in the social scale – a temporary return to the affluence they had enjoyed when they first married – for their new home, Redstone Manor, was an extensive house surrounded by fine gardens and woodland. This sudden ascent was thanks to Margery's brother Bob who, because he was not physically eligible for military service, had turned his outstanding talent as an entrepreneur to other aspects of the war effort, with very lucrative results. His parents were thus able to live in style – for a few years.

Bob Blackie, Margery's adored eldest brother, was a colourful character. He was a very good shot, and staged lavish shooting parties in a rented country house in Norfolk, Necton Hall (which has since been demolished). Tall and good-looking, he was full of zest and had gallant ways; he has been described by one who knew him as 'an irresponsible bachelor, a philanderer, who ran through fortunes and ended up broke, a speculator who was either living in extravagant luxury and giving lunch parties at the Ritz, or else was penniless'.

It is not surprising therefore that the Redstone ménage, under Bob's auspices, did not endure very long. After a few years the estate was sold to a developer, several hundred small houses were built in the grounds, and the big house was demolished. But it had been a blessing for Margery and her brothers and sisters that there had been, even for a short time, such a centre as Redstone Manor. The war had scattered the family; four of Margery's five brothers had served in the Army and all her sisters had been away from home (three had married during the war). But occasionally they had been able to forgather, and Redhill had provided the setting for a number of happy reunions.

After Redstone Manor was abandoned Margery moved to London, to live with her only unmarried sister Katharine ('Kay') in South Kensington. Kay, who was old enough to be her mother, had a flat in Harrington Road, which immediately adjoins Thurloe Street, and thus for the first time Margery came to know the part of London which was later to be her home ground for so many years, indeed for most of her life as a practising homoeopath. Sharing a flat with Kay was not an entirely congenial experience because, like her mother, she was a dominating personality, and she felt it her duty to look after her young sister. An ardent convert to the Church of England, Kay's piety was of the strict and aggressive kind – behind her back she was known in the family as 'the Dragon'.

When Margery's daily commuting began, in October 1917, the School of Medicine for Women was housed in an imposing red-brick complex in Hunter Street, centring round a court-yard known as 'the Quad', and the scale of the establishment can be judged by the fact that Margery was one of more than a hundred new arrivals, which brought the total number of students up to about four hundred and fifty. At this time the prospects for young women who wanted to enter the medical profession were newly encouraging; women doctors had been proving their worth during the war, and there was a much increased demand for their services. To provide for a great influx of students the school premises had been expanded and there were several new laboratories.

The beginning of each academic year was marked by an inaugural address, usually by a personality distinguished in the world of medicine. The aim was to give the newcomers some idea of the ethics of the medical profession, as well as guide-lines for organising their lives as students. They were told that they must not let their studies cut them off from other interests. 'Remember', said one of the speakers in Margery's time (perhaps reminding her of Miss Gilliland) 'that you will not reach anything like your ideal of being an efficient and useful doctor unless you know something of the world you and your patients live in . . . You must read widely and keep in touch with current politics, current literature and art and municipal life.' There was also a mention of behaviour and appearance. 'You must remember the importance of good manners and suitable and pretty clothes.' Here, in the emphasis on good manners, was an echo of a famous saying of Dr Elizabeth Garrett Anderson, that vehement campaigner for the recognition of women in medicine, who had been Dean of the School and later its President. 'The first thing women must learn', she once declared, 'is to behave like gentlemen.'

In Margery's time the Dean of the School was Louisa Aldrich Blake, the first woman to become a Master in Surgery (she was later created DBE). A true leader, she was regarded with much admiration by her students. Orpen's portrait shows a tall, well-built woman with looks that have been likened to those of Ingrid Bergman. According to one who knew her she had 'a quiet integrity and great courage', and she was also a perfectionist – 'everything had to be of the best'. She set high standards not only as Dean but as an athlete; she herself shone at cricket and was also a good horsewoman.

Another dominant figure on the staff with whom Margery was acquainted – relationships between the staff and the students were much more personal in those days than they are now – was Professor Winifred Cullis, renowned for the versatility of her medical interests as well as for her work as a professor of physiology.

Among her own contemporaries, Margery's best friend was a fellow student named Susanna Bernard, a tall, slim, serenely beautiful girl who later practised as a doctor in the Far East. Many of the young women who trained in the earlier days of the School hoped to devote themselves to a life of service abroad by becoming missionary doctors, but there is

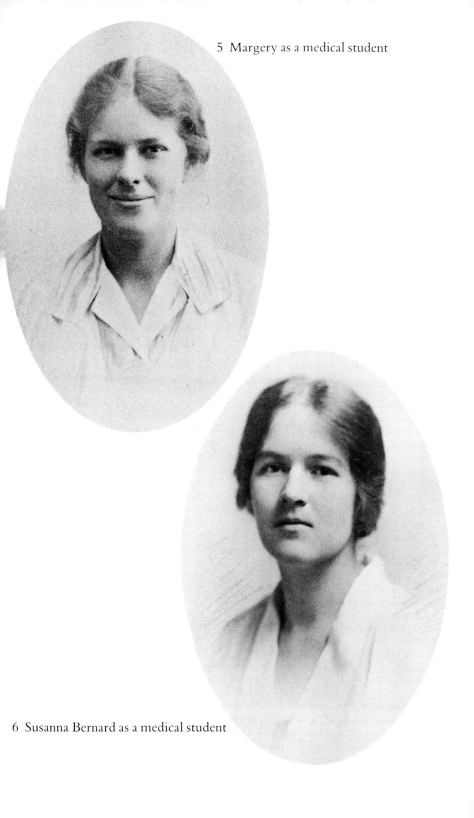

5 Margery as a medical student

6 Susanna Bernard as a medical student

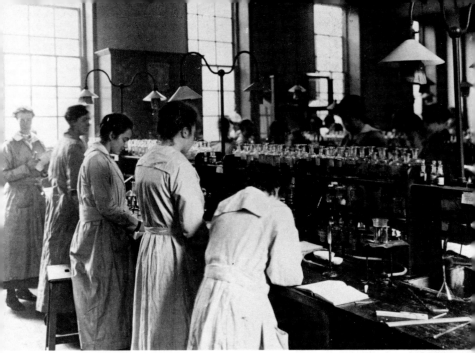

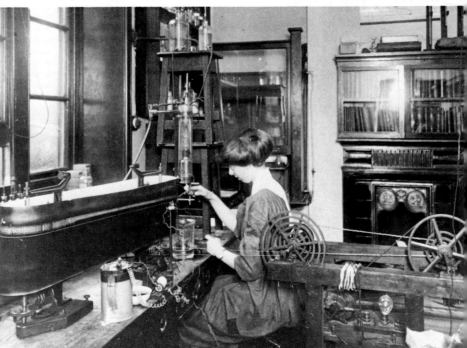

7 Students in the Old Chemistry Lab at the London School of Medicine for Women

8 One of the staff doing an experiment in physiology in the Old Physics Lab

no evidence that Margery herself was drawn towards missionary work while a student. She did however take on voluntary
social work in the East End at this time.

For her first years at the School Margery concentrated on the
three basic medical studies, Biology, Physics and Inorganic
Chemistry. A conscientious student, she was successful when
she sat for her first medical examination in July 1918, and
again, when she took Part I of her second medical examination
in the following March, she managed to pass. But examinations were not her forte. At the end of her third year, in March
1920, she failed when she took Part II of her second medical
examination. This was no disgrace however; students who
failed on a first attempt were normally given a second chance,
and when she tried again four months later she succeeded in
getting through.

There was little time in her life for anything but work,
although we know that one summer she and another girl went
hop-picking together – such outdoor vacation work was
encouraged by the Students' Union, which in those days
served primarily as a social centre. Within it a great number of
societies flourished, supported by enthusiasts for every kind of
activity and interest, from debating to hockey, from literature
to fencing. But Margery's dedication to her chosen study was
single-minded and the only time her name appears in the
School magazine is in connection with medicine; in 1922 she
became Secretary of the Union's Medical Society. During her
secretaryship the society held six meetings, with lectures by
expert speakers, and the subjects of these lectures are of some
interest, since Margery must have given serious thought to
them. They were as follows: 'Neurasthenia and Anxiety
Neuroses', 'Plastic Surgery of the Face', 'The Intracytoplas-
mic tubular system and the Thyroid Gland', 'Haematuria
[blood in the urine]', and 'The Criminal Court and the Medical Witness'. For this last lecture the speaker was Dr Bernard
Spilsbury, who was then on the staff of the school – this was

shortly before he was knighted for his work in forensic medicine.

From 1922 onwards the prospect of two sets of final examinations dominated Margery's life, for she aimed at gaining qualifications both from the University of London and from the Royal Colleges of England. So the next few years were years of intensive, exhausting work, focused on her clinical studies.

The first of the final examinations that she passed, in October 1922, was a College examination in Midwifery. Then in January 1923 she took her second College examination, in Medicine, and again succeeded in passing, thus becoming a Licentiate of the Royal College of Physicians (LRCP). And in July, at a second try, she passed the similar examination in Surgery, which made her a member of the Royal College of Surgeons (MRCS). These two examinations were commonly regarded as 'dummy runs' in preparation for the London University finals which would follow soon afterwards. Yet they had an important significance in themselves, for students who passed them thereby became registered medical practitioners, enabled to embark on professional work. Indeed some students chose to practise throughout their careers with College qualifications only.

In October 1923 Margery sat for her University of London finals for the first time – stiff tests in Medicine, Surgery and Obstetrics. She failed in all three subjects. There is no doubt that she was not a brilliant student of the prize-winning type, but she made up for this by her perseverance. With dogged determination she tried again and again. And eventually, in May 1926, she attained her goal. Thenceforth Dr Margery Blackie had the right to put after her name the letters MB (Bachelor of Medicine) and BS (Bachelor of Surgery).

Two years before she actually graduated, however, on the strength of her College qualifications, she had taken a step which was to decide the direction of her entire professional life. In April 1924 she had become a Resident at the London

Homoeopathic Hospital.* So there was an overlap between her earliest work in homoeopathy and the final stage of her non-homoeopathic training.

Here an important question arises. What was her attitude towards homoeopathy during her years as a student? Long afterwards she herself, on several occasions, made remarks which answer this question by reflecting her own experience. They show that she knew quite a lot about homoeopathy, and was strongly inclined towards it, even while she was being indoctrinated in general medicine, immersed in an atmosphere of scornful disbelief in the homoeopathic method. In one of her lectures she mentioned that while still a medical student she had been allowed to attend an out-patient clinic at the London Homoeopathic Hospital, and this had instilled in her a belief that while there is life, and the indicated homoeopathic remedy, there is more than hope, there is almost certainty. 'In my teaching hospital,' she said on another occasion, 'when I saw patients dying, I didn't have the satisfaction that the others had of believing that everything possible had been done. I felt they hadn't had the only thing that might have cured them.' Then she went on to say, 'I know that some people think that a student should be allowed to qualify before listening to anything about homoeopathy but I disagree. If he knows something of it as a student he can compare the two systems during these years and that saves a lot of time. Then, when he decides to investigate homoeopathy further he can go straight ahead.' She considered that she herself had been very lucky in having 'a slight homoeopathic knowledge' while studying medicine.

Another time she related an anecdote which not only confirmed her own attitude – as a student – towards homoeopathy, but also showed that the prejudice against it among the teaching staff at the Royal Free Hospital was not as unanimous as one might have expected. 'I was interested in homoeopathy before I started my medical training,' she said, 'and on a ward round one day in my teaching hospital the chief asked what I

* It did not become the *Royal* London Homoeopathic Hospital until 1948.

would prescribe for a patient. Whether I forgot where I was, or whether it was bravado, I know not, but I replied "*Nux vomica*".★ My friends grew pale with fright, but nothing happened. Passing me in the corridor later he stopped and said "A very good idea. I always carry it", and pulled from his waistcoat pocket two small bottles of pills – one *Nux vomica* and the other *Carbo veg.*'.†

★ This homoeopathic remedy is prepared from the seeds of the fruit of an Asiatic tree. Strychnine is derived from the same source.
† *Carbo vegetabilis*, a homoeopathic remedy prepared from wood charcoal.

Hospital Physician

At twenty-six Margery was a spirited young woman, courageous and boldly independent in outlook. When she took the plunge into the world of homoeopathy, when she became a house physician at the London Homoeopathic Hospital in Great Ormond Street, she took a plunge into a man's world; after living hitherto in a world of women she suddenly became one of a very small minority in a hospital staffed almost entirely by men.

She showed courage, too, in embracing homoeopathy, for she did so with certain reservations. Later on, looking back to this stage of her career, she admitted – time and again – that despite the confidence in homoeopathic medicine she had always felt, she had made up her mind that she would not commit herself blindly. By means of working at the hospital and by intensive study she meant to find out for herself whether the claims that were made for it were valid – a fascinating echo! This was precisely the attitude taken up long ago by her uncle, the great Dr Compton Burnett, when he first resolved to put homoeopathy to the test 'at the bedside'.

The setting for Margery's brave experiment was not the building where the London Homoeopathic Hospital was first established. Golden Square was the original site where it was founded in 1849 by Dr Frederick Quin, famed as a brilliant disciple of Hahnemann's. In the late 1830s Quin had been the first man to introduce homoeopathy to Britain, and his importance can hardly be exaggerated. Not only a talented doctor but a man of acute intelligence and charm (he was reputed to be the illegitimate son of a duchess) he followed up the founding of the hospital by launching the British Homoeopathic Society. The aim of this learned society was to promote the study and understanding of the whole subject, and to ensure the maintaining of high professional standards.

Spurned and derided by the medical establishment, the little hospital in Golden Square, with only twenty-five beds, achieved striking successes during the cholera epidemic of 1854. Indeed the figures were so startling (only 16.4 per cent deaths against the average of 51 per cent in other hospitals) that the enemies of homoeopathy tried – unsuccessfully – to suppress them. Soon the need to expand the hospital became urgent and it was moved to premises in Great Ormond Street which allowed for fifty beds. But even this did not anything like meet the demand for homoeopathic treatment at the end of the nineteenth century, and in 1893 the foundation stone of a much larger hospital, at the corner of Great Ormond Street and Queen Square, was laid by Princess Mary, Duchess of Teck, accompanied by her daughter 'Princess May', later Queen Mary.

Homoeopathy has long attracted adherents from among the aristocracy (perhaps because of its concentration upon the individual person – it is the antithesis of mass production) and its association with the royal family was no flash in the pan; throughout its history in England there have been close links with royalty.

When Margery was first at the hospital its Patron was Edward Prince of Wales, while the President was the Duke of York who later, as King George VI, was to give the hospital the title of 'Royal'. (Furthermore he named one of his racehorses 'Hypericum' after a homoeopathic remedy which had helped him. Hypericum, a bay mare, was winner of the Thousand Guineas Stakes at Newmarket in 1946.) Earlier, the Prince of Wales's association with homoeopathy had been illustrated by the appointment of Dr John Weir, the eminent homoeopath, as a Physician-in-Ordinary in 1923, and by his subsequent knighthood in 1932.

Before this the royal dependence on homoeopathy had been unofficial, though no secret. Queen Alexandra's favourite doctor was a homoeopath, Dr George Moore. And earlier still Prince Leopold of the Belgians, Queen Victoria's uncle, had been a patient of Dr Quin's; while Queen Adelaide, the German wife of King William IV, had been attended by Hahnemann's favourite pupil, Dr Johann Stapf.

During the course of the nineteenth century various distinguished public figures also underwent 'the Hahnemann treatment', or experimented for themselves with what might be called homoeopathic first aid. In diplomatic circles, both in London and on the continent, homoeopathy was much talked of. It had been banned in Austria by the powerful medical establishment so it was a controversial topic. But Quin was consulted by many eminent personages including the Marquess of Anglesey, who some years after he lost a leg at Waterloo developed a distressing nervous complaint, the *tic douloureux*. Another nobleman, who suffered from 'facial neuralgia' and who turned to homoeopathy – in fact he turned to Hahnemann himself, for 'the Master' was based in Paris at the time – was the seventh Earl of Elgin, who, after his final battles on behalf of the Parthenon marbles, lived his last sad years in France. It is on record that Elgin tried to persuade others to try 'the Hahnemann treatment'.

Then in the 1850s, Robert Browning became a convert. There is an interesting passage in one of the letters written by Elizabeth Barrett Browning to her sister from Florence in March 1858 which describes how he was won over.

> Everybody has bad influenza; and Robert was so exceedingly unwell that he was persuaded to try homoeopathy. He submitted, with a smile of scorn, to give it a fair trial. By degrees the scorn disappeared – there seemed 'really something in it' – undeniably he 'felt better'. Now he has a regular healthy appetite . . . He takes the globules in water, which is now considered the strongest

form. Certainly the medicine takes hold of the constitution. I would not trust to it where a rapid *shock* to the system is necessary (as in the case of sudden inflammation or fever), but in any chronic affection I really *would*. We are going to buy bottles and a book, so as to have our fate in our own hands – so far.

Disraeli, during his final years, when he was suffering from persistent attacks of gout, bronchitis and asthma, found that Dr Joseph Kidd, the leading British homoeopath of the day, was the only physician able to help him. 'I entertain the highest opinion of Dr Kidd', he wrote to his friend, the Countess of Bradford, in 1877. 'All the medical men I have known, and I have seen some of the highest, seem much inferior to him.' This preference for Dr Kidd became suddenly a matter of embarrassment at the time of Disraeli's last illness, for Queen Victoria, in her anxiety, urged that a second opinion, from a non-homoeopathic doctor, should be obtained. Sir William Jenner, who was first asked to help, excused himself on grounds that it would be a breach of professional conduct to consult with 'an irregular'. Next to be summoned was Dr Richard Quain, and he – after initial hesitation – agreed to join in consultation with Dr Kidd, though this earned him heated accusations of violating professional ethics.

The monumental red-brick building on the corner of Great Ormond Street and Queen Square, which throughout Margery's time represented the main stronghold of homoeopathy in Britain, looks externally very much the same today as when she first entered its doors. But latterly, within it, there have been many changes and its original character has been lost.* When she started work there in April 1924 it was exclusively homoeopathic, with the status of a general

*When the National Health Service was inaugurated in 1948 the hospital was one of those allowed to retain its autonomy, with its own management committee. Thus its original ethos could be retained. After the 1974 reorganisation of the N H S, however, the management committees of all hospitals other than postgraduate teaching hospitals were disbanded. Thereafter began a steady decline in the hospital's morale.

hospital supported by voluntary contributions. This meant of course a constant struggle to make ends meet, for the hospital had been founded to provide for the needs of the poor, and many of the patients were treated entirely free; others contributed financially according to their means. But it also meant that the atmosphere was one of dedication and enthusiasm. A contemporary of Margery's has recalled that when he started at the hospital he was struck by two outstanding things, its quietness and its leisurely air. 'I soon found that it was run for the sake of the patients and not for noisy students and rather harassed doctors.'

So from the very beginning of her 'apprenticeship' Margery's working life was permeated by an attitude of devotion which she shared with all her fellow physicians, including the senior consultant, Dr John Henry Clarke. Clarke, in his day, was the hospital's revered elder statesman – he had joined the staff in 1881. One of the greatest experts of his time on the subject of homoeopathic medicines, he was internationally renowned. Margery had a felicitous personal link with him because he had known and greatly admired her uncle, and he several times did her the honour of inviting her to accompany him to the Royal Society of Medicine.

Dr Clarke was, like her uncle, an energetic controversialist, as witnessed by his paper 'The Two Paths in Homoeopathy', for there were – and still are – two rival schools of thought as to how homoeopathy should be presented to the world at large. Clarke, like Compton Burnett, was an ardent upholder of the clinical approach; he insisted that results must be allowed to speak for themselves. Compton Burnett's main opponent had been another eminent homoeopath, Dr Richard Hughes, whose ambition was to convert the unbelievers by giving them scientific evidence 'so codified and purged of extraneous detail as to be irrefutable on any objective reading'. To Hughes, Compton Burnett's lack of scientific method, his chatty tone, his resolute reliance on the clinical, and his defiantly popularising approach had been anathema. Meanwhile

Compton Burnett, with gusto, had denounced Hughes as a timid dreamer, and his views as dangerously restrictive. No doubt Margery, when she was escorted by Dr Clarke to the Royal Society of Medicine, heard some persuasive advocacy of her uncle's beliefs.

Margery's two 'chiefs', the two physicians with whom she was constantly in touch during her years as a Resident, and whose lectures she eagerly attended, were doctors of exceptional calibre. Later she often paid tribute to 'these two wonderful men', Douglas Borland and Charles Wheeler, who by their teaching, and by their examples in diagnosis and prescribing, set standards which remained with her all her life. Both men influenced her profoundly. Dr Wheeler, the senior of the two, was a man of great intellectual brilliance who hailed from Australia. Dedicated to his work in medicine, he also had wide-ranging interests in art, music, drama, literature and science. A kind man, genial and tolerant, he delighted in sharing his very extensive knowledge with beginners who, like Margery, were really keen to learn. He liked to start his rounds very early and always arrived half an hour beforehand so as to have breakfast with his house physician. Thus she had frequent opportunities, over tea and toast, to learn from him about homoeopathic medicines, where they come from, who had discovered them, how they should be prescribed and so on. 'The spoken word in homoeopathy', she once said, 'is worth pages of printed ones'.

But it was Dr Borland who counted for most – by far the most. Writing of him after his death Margery called him 'a giant among doctors'. He was 'a born doctor', she said, and eminently suited to be a homoeopath, because he was always interested in the whole person – body, mind and spirit, so much so that there had been a time when he was undecided whether to go into the Church or into medicine. At a first meeting Dr Borland, who was a Scot from Glasgow, often gave an impression of aloofness. With his unhurried walk and impeccable suits, his amused drawl and what has been called 'the veiled touch of mild and kindly sarcasm' in his talk, he seemed an imperturbable man of the world. But all this was only a mask for his shyness; behind it there was an utterly charming, gentle and generous personality. He was also, however, a man whose intensive dedication to his work took an inevitable toll – off duty he was a chain-smoker.

If a Resident was willing to work and anxious to learn, Borland took endless pains to teach, and his rounds were always full of information. In 1924 he was the hospital's physician for the diseases of children; in addition to his work in the wards he had a busy clinic for the young out-patients who crowded in with their mothers every Monday morning. Perhaps Margery learnt most from him by sitting in on these out-patient clinics. She and another young house surgeon, Dr Frank Bodman, who was her exact contemporary at the hospital and who was to become her lifelong friend, always made a point of being there while Dr Borland took his cases. And from then on, so Margery later declared, she was certain that in order to learn homoeopathy it is essential to see cases taken by experienced seniors.

She once gave an account of Dr Borland's clinical methods which is of special interest since it reflects the methods that later characterised her own approach. 'He had a marvellous gift of never seeming to be in a hurry,' she said. 'He might have a notice on the desk saying "five new and sixty old patients", but each patient left feeling that he or she was the one he was really interested in; he had listened to everything they had to say, and understood. It was an education in itself to hear him take a history. He seldom if ever asked direct questions, but got the answers he wanted by various means.' He seemed to know instinctively what type of person he was dealing with, from their appearance, their entering, the way they sat down and started to talk. 'In certain cases it only needed a few sympathetic, understanding words and the whole story poured forth. To another type he might pretend to misunderstand what they meant, or make a remark that annoyed, and again he would get the story.'

Margery found that one of the best ways of learning from Dr Borland and Dr Wheeler was by informal chats over coffee after their ward rounds. 'We put up our problems, and they gave us their opinions and experiences and advice about the drugs to read up and compare.'

Of course Margery had to 'read up and compare' very extensively, and a precious relic of her studies has survived, a tiny loose-leaf notebook, obviously much used, containing the notes she made during her earliest years as a doctor. In a minute hand, on page after page, are listed the main substances used in homoeopathy (many of them, but by no means all, of herbal origin), *Aconite*, *Belladonna* (deadly nightshade) and so on, with descriptions under each heading, in great detail, of the symptoms, both physical and mental, caused by *large* doses of the substance in healthy persons. She listed these symptoms under subject headings such as Appearance, Mouth and Teeth, Throat, Appetite, Respiratory, Heart, Sleep, Mind, Eyes, etc. And the purpose of this record was to arrive at what homoeopaths call 'drug pictures', so that she would realise at once, when at a consultation she recognised various symptoms or characteristics in a patient, which 'drug picture' they indicated, and therefore which medicine (in a *very small* dosage) she ought to prescribe.

As we know, Margery was already familiar with the basic principle of homoeopathy, that like must be treated by like. She knew for instance that the homoeopathic medicine *Arsenicum album*, which is prepared from white arsenic, the well-known poison, can be used very effectively – in minute quantities – to treat acute bacterial food poisoning. But she needed to come to grips, little by little, with the endless knowledge needed to implement Hahnemann's axiom to the full. And the essential first step was to memorise the most important drug pictures. (Her uncle, she once said, began by knowing ten drug pictures very thoroughly before he started prescribing. He claimed that if a beginner knows ten drug pictures like that he will be able to prescribe well for a good many cases he meets in a day.) Margery's entries in her little notebook can therefore be regarded as the basis of all her future work as a homoeopath. To illustrate the style of her record, here are some of her notes under the heading GELSEMIUM (this remedy, derived from yellow jasmine, is often very effective at the early stages of influenza).

> GENERAL Aching of back and limbs – v. bad. Weary all over. Headache affects vision. Flu beginning with nasal discharge. V. sorry for himself. Headache and pain.
> THROAT V. painful. Slight ulceration. Swelling. Redness . . . Spasm in throat on swallowing.
> MENTALITY Resents being disturbed. Wants to be left alone. Sees things. V. often sleepless for hours. Distressed and uncomfortable. Lies absolutely still; no tossing about. V. emotional.

The concept of the drug picture was a vital part of Margery's clinical training, and here Dr Borland was her mentor-in-chief. On his ward rounds he would stop beside the bed of a very ill child or some other patient and remain silent for a minute or two. Then, having examined the patient, he would first ask Margery what she wanted to give, and afterwards tell her what he was sure the patient needed. As he was leaving the ward he would often pause at the door to say, 'Go back and look at that patient several times today. Get him into your head.' That particular patient, he said, was the perfect example of such and such a drug picture.

Margery, as a Resident, often had to take full responsibility for prescribing without Dr Borland's support, as is shown by a fragmentary piece of evidence, a personal testimony, from the sister of one of her patients at this time. On 2 June 1924 (this was only two months after Margery started work at the hospital) a boy of twelve was taken to the homoeopathic dispensary at Shepherd's Bush and pneumonia was diagnosed. He was thereupon rushed to Great Ormond Street and admitted to the Hahnemann Ward. 'He was seen by Dr Blackie,' his sister has recently written, 'who prescribed a homoeopathic remedy, which was considered to have saved his life' (this was, of course, years before antibiotics).

Evidently Margery was already beginning to show her flair for diagnosis; she was learning that perception of the totality of a patient's characteristics, both of body and mind, not only his pathological symptoms, is vital to the homoeopath's task – even in cases of emergency. Two cases of pneumonia might need to be treated with two quite different remedies. The whole biological picture had to be taken into account. This diagnostic approach soon became second nature to her, and looking back to those early days she often smiled to remember an occasion when she went to a theatre with Frank Bodman. The play was *Hedda Gabler*, and the two young doctors had immense fun identifying the characteristics of the various actors and actresses and 'prescribing' for them, as well as for some of the members of the audience. 'We were quite amazed at the number of counterparts we had in practice as patients.'*

During this initial stage of Margery's medical career, while she was still only a Resident at the hospital, a learner as regards homoeopathy, she was already taking her first steps as a teacher, the role in which, later in life, she was so pre-eminent. This came about because immediately next door to the hospital there was a missionary medical school which had close links with homoeopathy. The Missionary School of Medicine had been founded in 1903, and in the 1920s it was still a flourishing concern, preparing students for service in remote areas

* There is an amusing echo of this 'game' in an article which appeared in 1947 in the *British Homoeopathic Journal*. A certain Dr A. C. G. Ross, who since his youth had been an admirer of Dr Johnson, had gathered together a wealth of evidence about the great man's characteristics, both physical and mental – his indolence, capricious appetite, uncontrollable drinking of tea, love of fat, untidiness, fearfulness of hell-fire, dislike of clean linen etc. etc. And he had found that all these symptoms coincided with the drug picture of the homoeopathic medicine *Sulphur*. 'No doubt if he had been given *Sulphur* he might have worn a clean shirt more often', Dr Ross concluded, 'and been healthier and happier, but he could scarcely have been better loved by his friends.'

throughout the world. The object of the school was not to train and send out medical missionaries as such, but to equip young men and women (who had been training in Protestant Bible Colleges) with a knowledge of elementary medicine and allied subjects. This was to prepare them for emergencies among the people of their areas, and also for taking care of their own health and that of their fellow missionaries.

Many medical subjects were included in the school's short courses but homoeopathic principles and practice were dominant, and in order to see clinical work in progress the students attended the hospital's wards and out-patient departments. We have no details of Margery's earliest teaching work, but we know that she began it during her second year at the hospital, 1925, for that was when her name first appeared in the list of the school's teaching staff. And it is notable that the list includes all the leading physicians at the hospital: Borland, Wheeler, Weir, McCrae, Rorke, and many others.

This was the beginning of a long-standing connection between Margery and the Missionary School of Medicine, which appealed to her especially because of its spirit of Christian service.*

As a resident doctor at the hospital Margery had to spend most of her life on the spot. But off duty she was now living her own life, no longer under the governessy eye of her sister Kay. Instead she was sharing a flat near Baker Street, at 66 George Street, with her friend Susanna Bernard, who had qualified just before her and was now embarking upon a career in medicine at the Royal Free Hospital. The two got on well together, and when 'Sue' moved to the house of her aunt Mrs McWilliam in Drayton Gardens, Margery moved with her; in all they lived together for about six years.

At this time there was a serious disappointment for

---

* This connection still continues, for in 1982 a biennial prize for homoeopathy, in memory of Dr Margery Blackie, was established within the school.

Margery, an abortive romance. She fell in love with a young man who had a passion for music – they used to go to promenade concerts together, and evidently Margery was seriously smitten, for she had hopes of marriage. Her family however disapproved, for what reasons we do not know, and they even employed detectives to trail her suitor, to obtain evidence that would persuade Margery to give him up. This sad episode finally ended when he married someone else, and in later life Margery very seldom spoke of it, though she once said to a friend, 'Music – that's the one thing I'm grateful to him for.'

In the background of her life there had been various developments in the Blackie family. Her brother Frank, who since the age of nineteen had been working in India, had returned to England after the First World War and taken up farming in Norfolk. So it is not surprising that Margery's parents, after Redstone Manor was sold, decided to move to West Norfolk, where their new home was at Downham Market, then the main market town for an extensive farming area as well as a thriving centre of Methodism. At Trafalgar House, Downham Market, Robert and Lizzie Blackie settled down at last, and there happiness came to them – but also grief. At Trafalgar House they celebrated their golden wedding, but in the Downham Market cemetery there is a tombstone commemorating the deaths of two of Margery's brothers, both young bachelors. Avery had died in India in 1925 and Alan, Margery's favourite brother after Bob, was killed in a French railway accident in 1927.

Into Partnership

Before Margery had completed her novitiate – her time as a hospital Resident, when she was in turn house surgeon, house physician, and casualty officer – her reservations concerning homoeopathy had vanished and she was setting her sights more and more towards the aim of starting a practice of her own. This ambition was spurred by the encouragement of her closest friend in the hospital, Dr Helena Banks, a young Scotswoman of the same age as herself, who was later to become her partner in practice and one of her most devoted intimates. Dr Banks had started work at Great Ormond Street slightly later than Margery – she became gynaecology and casualty house surgeon in the autumn of 1924 – but very soon, like Margery, she was yearning to have her own practice. She did, in fact, succeed in starting up a homoeopathic practice in south-east London, in Lewisham, as soon as her time as a Resident was up.

The most compelling influence upon Margery however was the example of Dr Borland, her adored master, who like the other leading homoeopaths she knew combined his specialised hospital work with a general practice in the West End (he had consulting rooms in Devonshire Place). So when he gladly gave her a plan for working a practice and encouraged her to take the plunge, she resolved to go ahead. No doubt he also offered to help by sending her patients.

So it was in 1926, a few months after the General Strike, that Margery, at twenty-eight, 'put up her plate' outside number 10 Drayton Gardens, the large terrace house on the borders of

Kensington and Fulham which belonged to Susanna Bernard's aunt; it was at that time Margery's London home. Proudly, after her name, she was now able to add the letters MB (Bachelor of Medicine) and BS (Bachelor of Surgery) for at last, after several failures, she had succeeded, earlier that year, in passing her final examinations.

But the house in Drayton Gardens was not her only professional address. In the *British Homoeopathic Journal* for 1926–7 the following notice appeared: 'Dr Marjory [*sic*] G. Blackie has begun practice at 10 Drayton Gardens, S.W.10 and 68 Fulham Road, S.W.3.'

There is a fascinating story of how she acquired her second foothold. On the day after she put up her plate in Drayton Gardens she decided to take a look at the surrounding district. Turning into the Fulham Road and making her way northwards, in the direction of the area near Harrington Road which she already knew well, she had just passed the Cancer Hospital (now the Royal Marsden) when she happened to notice, on the left, a chemist's shop. Number 68 Fulham Road looks very different now; its façade has been completely redesigned and the shop is part of an Italian boutique for men's fashions. But sixty years ago it belonged to one of the few homoeopathic chemists in central London, Headland & Co., and Margery's eye was caught by a painted-out sign which was still just legible: 'Homoeopathic Dispensary, Mondays, Wednesdays and Fridays'. Much intrigued she questioned the chemist who told her that the dispensary had been closed for twelve years. 'What about opening it again?' she asked. The chemist was a friendly man and without hesitation he showed her two rooms on the first floor. 'They'll do splendidly,' she said, 'and I'd like to start next Monday.' At the weekend she herself papered the future consulting room and arranged for some furniture to be sent in. Meanwhile the chemist and his assistant prepared the waiting room. Word soon got round that the dispensary was being reopened, and when Margery arrived on the Monday she found a dozen patients waiting for her.

So now she was on her own! Without any senior physician at hand, without – at first – any partner to share her work and her problems, she had to judge every case and decide on every prescription entirely from her own knowledge and intuition.

One of her first cases was a dramatic one which she never forgot. The patient was a boy of eighteen, diffident, undecided, embarrassed, who came in with his mother. He was absolutely bald, with no eyelashes or eyebrows. Margery took his history and discovered, among other things, that his eating habits were very abnormal. Although he was often hungry he would only eat half a plateful at a time, and then in less than an hour he wanted more. He also had a craving for sweet things, so in order to make him eat, his mother used to cover his meat with jam. From these and other symptoms, including his lack of hair, Margery recognised his drug picture, and realised that the medicine he needed was *Lycopodium* (a remedy derived from club moss). She prescribed accordingly, and when he came back a month later he had 'a little mat of hair all over his head'. There was then a slightly disconcerting sequel. To Margery's dismay her delighted patient sent friend after friend, including an old man who had been bald for years, in the hopes that she would give them courses of *Lycopodium* with equally spectacular results. How could the poor young man have known that in homoeopathy one can never generalise? Each patient is a unique person, and two people who are suffering from the same trouble may present entirely different drug pictures, and thus have to be treated quite differently, except in the case of various common ailments or emergencies where certain homoeopathic remedies may be regarded as first aid, for example *Arnica* (leopard's bane) for shock and bruises, *Rhus toxicodendron* (poison ivy) for muscular pains, *Hypericum* (St John's wort) for cuts or wounds.

In contrast to the hairless young man, some of Margery's earliest private patients were long-time devotees of homoeopathy, who were so proud of their amateur knowledge that they sometimes prompted her. For them Richard Hughes,

that great homoeopath of the previous generation, was a
magic name. They all had their little chests of remedies and
they often told Margery that she had better prescribe such and
such a medicine 'because Dr Hughes had advised it'.

Margery soon learnt how to conduct her consultations. She
followed Dr Borland's method of keeping as quiet as possible.
The patient, she once said – she was speaking of women –
must be allowed to tell her story in her own way. She will tell
you strange facts that she thinks have nothing to do with her
complaints, but often, seemingly by chance, you thus get very
important indications. Such an opportunity to talk at length to
someone who is really keen to hear is, in fact, from the
patient's point of view, one of the great attractions of a
consultation with a homoeopathic doctor. 'A new patient is
often encouraged because this is the first time a doctor has
listened to her and encouraged her to talk about her strange
symptom.'

Little by little Margery developed the consulting-room
methods that in course of time became second nature to her.
'The taking of the history is not merely the collecting of facts,'
she once said. 'Those sheets of questions with a space for an
answer which I used as a Resident are not good.' But there
were of course questions that had to be asked, and some of
them, to the uninitiated patient, must undoubtedly have seemed
to bear no relation whatever to the main trouble. But as a
homoeopath Margery needed to get to know the whole person, not only his past history, and any tendencies to hereditary
or latent diseases; she had to find out what his habits were,
both physical and mental. His eating and drinking habits were
specially important. Was his appetite good? Had it varied
recently? Did any food upset him? Did he dislike something
particularly? Had he a special craving for sweets, or salt, or
spicy foods? Was he thirsty? For hot or cold drinks? And how
much at a time? A full glass at one go or just a few sips?

It must be added that Margery's homoeopathic approach
did not exclude the forms of investigation which are common

to every branch of practising medicine – pathological tests, X-ray examinations, blood-pressure checks and so on; these were sometimes essential, though she tried to keep them to a minimum. Nevertheless she had to unlearn one of the basic principles that had been drummed into her as a medical student. She had been told, again and again, that the primary purpose of a consultation is to identify the patient's disease, and then to determine which of his organs are affected, and how far they are involved. The aim of the homoeopathic consultation, on the other hand, is to establish how a given morbid condition has developed *in the person who has come for help*, to explore the evolution of the disease in that particular person. This is why Margery, when towards the end of her life she wrote a book about homoeopathy, entitled it *The Patient, Not the Cure*.

So first of all comes the clinical diagnosis and the recognition of the patient's drug picture, with the consequent identification of the medicine appropriate to the person concerned.★ Then comes the actual prescribing and here the choice of the appropriate medicine is not the only immediate decision to be made. The homoeopathic doctor, when deciding which medicine to prescribe, also has to decide what 'potency' of the remedy to specify. 'Potency' . . . In the context of homoeopathic medicine what does this word mean? Hahnemann defined a potency as a 'power'. But more explicitly this important term means the energy hitherto latent in a substance – whether in an active or in an inert state – which has been brought out by a special mode of preparation, dependent upon the skills of the homoeopathic pharmacist. This mode of preparation – 'potentising' or 'dynamisation' – consists of a carefully controlled process of serial dilutions alternated with

★In strictly homoeopathic usage, a patient's condition – his drug picture – is named according to the indicated remedy rather than according to his most evident symptoms, as identified by the clinical diagnosis, e.g., arthritis, though in conversation the homoeopath normally uses the familiar nomenclature.

'succussions' (vigorous shakings) which increase the 'dynamic energy' of the substance.

Hahnemann himself, after he discovered the paradox that the more often a medical substance is diluted the stronger are its effects, had further experimented by alternating dilutions and succussions in a definite arithmetical ratio, and he had found that this procedure released a hidden 'power', or 'potency', possessed by the medicine itself. He found too that in clinical practice there is a place for 'more power' or 'less power', and thus the concept of high potencies and low potencies came into being. These have ever since been the common coin of homoeopathy; the two interrelated principles of dilution and succussion have been the basis of homoeopathic pharmacology, despite the fact that no full explanation of the processes involved has yet been given in the language of science. No one has so far explained how or why these phenomena interact, but for the majority of homoeopaths the beneficent effects upon sick patients are all that matters.

This lack of 'scientific proof' as regards potencies is at the heart of the reservations which are still felt, at the present time, by many doctors brought up in the tradition of the medical schools. Margery, who in her early days was an ardent supporter of the empirical, under the influence of Dr Clarke and the teachings of her uncle, came round, towards the end of her career, to the viewpoint of Richard Hughes; in other words she became very much aware that in order to win over the medical establishment scientific 'proofs' would have to be given. One would have to be able to say, in terms of physics and chemistry and physiology, *'This is how homoeopathy works.'* And she herself took active steps to initiate the necessary research, as we shall see later.*

The question of the rival advantages of high and low potencies has always been, and still is, a matter of controversy

---

* Here, in passing, an impertinent suggestion comes to mind. Surely some earnest homoeopathic researcher ought to study the effects of succussion upon alcoholic tinctures as practised by means of cocktail shakers.

and heated debate among homoeopaths. In general terms, the lower potencies cause milder reactions and are the most suitable for homoeopathic first aid, or for long-term treatments, while the higher potencies are often more rapidly effective, but may at first cause 'aggravations', temporary intensifications of the disease symptoms, just as vaccination and other innoculations sometimes do.

Among the leading doctors at the hospital when Margery was beginning her career, several were firm believers in high-potency prescribing, especially Dr Borland, and even more so Dr John Weir (as he was then). They were two of the British homoeopaths who before the First World War had gone briefly to Chicago to study under the eminent Dr Kent, a committed exponent of high-potency prescribing, whose influence in America was dominant at the time. It has indeed persisted elsewhere and prescribers of high potencies are still sometimes referred to as 'Kentians'.

Convinced chiefly no doubt by Dr Borland, Margery was, in her early days, a keen upholder of Kentian principles. She once related that after a meeting of the British Homoeopathic Society (she became an associate member in 1926) there was a discussion on potencies – 'always an inflammable subject' – and the heat of the discussion went to her head. 'I remember vividly rising to my feet for the first time to express my opinions,' she later recalled. 'I implored the erring faction to give up their evil ways and use only high potencies! Dr Wheeler, who was in the chair, tried to pour oil on troubled waters, and no one could do it better than he. He remarked that most people learned to walk before they tried to run, but that the young today seemed to want to fly, straight from the cradle.'

But Margery was never entirely against low potencies. At the hospital she had witnessed how the potencies used by Dr Wheeler, for instance, were sometimes high, sometimes low. 'I did see a number of cases of pulmonary tuberculosis', she once admitted, 'treated entirely with low potencies, and could

not have asked for better results. I felt convinced that there was
a place for both high and low potencies but the question was –
what was the place for each?'

In 1926 she was, of course, still a beginner, as Dr Wheeler so
tactfully pointed out. Years later, with half a century of
diagnosis and prescribing behind her, she summed up her
views on potencies as follows: 'Since I've started gardening
I've compared my high potency to a shower of rain, and my
low potency to the watering can that I must use occasionally
on some corner of the garden in order to weather a critical
stage.'

Margery attained to senior status in the medical profession, by
becoming a Doctor of Medicine, when she was only thirty.
And it is notable that in July 1928, when she was awarded the
MD degree by the University of London, she was the only
woman candidate. Already it was being recognised that her
abilities were equal to those of men. Already she was emerg-
ing as a potential leader.

As she entered her thirties the pattern of her life was
changing, though as always it was dominated by single-
minded dedication to her work. Susanna Bernard had by now
started a non-homoeopathic practice of her own near Sloane
Square, prior to joining the Colonial Medical Service, and
before long, as Margery became more and more deeply
involved in homoeopathy, it was inevitable that their paths
should diverge. They still kept in touch, however, and were
affectionate friends; later, when Susanna married and had a
daughter, she asked Margery to be godmother.

Number 10 Drayton Gardens remained the official base of
Margery's practice until the end of the 1920s, but then a new
address for Dr Margery G. Blackie appeared in the *Medical
Directory*: 18 Alfred Place. This house, which later (when
Alfred Place was renamed) became number 18 Thurloe Street,
was to be Margery's London home for the rest of her life.

In the meantime, at the hospital, where she was now clinical

assistant to Dr Borland and was thus concentrating on children's diseases, her friendship with Helena Banks, then clinical assistant to Dr Rorke, the physician for nervous diseases,
was growing stronger. In February 1929 Margery was prom-
oted to be assistant physician in the children's department and
in this same year she and Helena decided to join forces and
embark on a joint practice at Alfred Place. Dr Banks gave up
her practice in Lewisham, and the two friends established
themselves together in the pleasant terrace house where
Margery was already practising.

Helena Banks, with her buxom figure, dark bobbed hair
and ready smile, was a very likeable person, by nature kind
and warm-hearted. She had a keen sense of humour and a great
sense of fun, while at the same time, according to one of her
patients, she was always 'delightfully straightforward and
downright'; she called a spade a spade so that everyone knew
exactly where they were with her. One of her friends, too,
remembers her bluntness and adds 'she was a Scot' – she had a
trace of a Scottish accent. In temperament she and Margery
complemented one another most happily and they were ideal
partners.

Dr Banks gradually acquired many patients of her own but
she often stood in for Margery, who once said of her that as a
doctor she had exceptional wisdom and judgement. But in
addition to her medical work she excelled in dealing with
business matters, keeping accounts, and drafting letters and
reports. The smooth running of the practice and also of the
house was entirely due to her. In Margery's own words 'she
kept my feet on the ground'. Yet although full of initiative and
ideas she was shy and retiring. She always worked in the
background, and wanted any credit to go to Margery and not
to herself.

Besides all this 'Banks' – as Margery usually called her – was
a very congenial companion and friend, with a sensitive,
artistic side. She had a special skill in arranging flowers, and a
patient of hers, who had likened her to the great Constance

Spry, once remarked that she had 'out-spryed Spry'. The beginning of her friendship with Margery had been when they were both hospital Residents and Margery happened to be briefly ill. Helena had brought a beautifully arranged bowl of flowers to her room, deposited it at the bedside and walked out again without a word.

Helena's background, like Margery's, was homoeopathic; her father had been a homoeopath who left Scotland to practise in the Midlands. Helena, after Cheltenham Ladies' College and Birmingham University, had worked in conventional medicine for a time, encouraged to do so by her father, who wanted her to find out for herself whether or not she was dissatisfied. So she and Margery had progressed along more or less the same road. And there was another, deeper bond between the two. They were both of them committed Christians and both came from strongly nonconformist families. Helena's paternal grandfather had been a Presbyterian minister.

To understand Margery Blackie it is essential to see her in the context of her evangelical faith, with its tradition of service to others, and of unquestioning dependence on the Bible. She herself was reticent as to her stance in the matter of religion; she did not regard herself as having a label. But we can deduce that here, as elsewhere, she relied on her womanly intuition. She was no theologian and she once said, 'you have to believe from the heart – the heart not the head'. At the same time the nonconformist ethos was deeply rooted in her. And although in her day medical students were no longer required to recite the Hippocratic Oath on graduation, Margery knew it well and took its guidelines as seriously as if she had actually made the vow (and as if Hippocrates himself had been a Christian). The declaration which had been the basis of medical ethics through the centuries gave a central purpose to the dedication of her life to helping others – to healing others.

I will use treatment to help the sick according to my ability and judgement but I will never use it to injure or wrong them . . . In purity and in holiness I will guard my life and my art . . . Now if I keep this oath and break it not, may I enjoy honour, in my life and art, among all men for all time, but if I transgress and forswear myself, may the opposite befall me.

Margery was certainly a committed Christian, yes, but in the early days of her practice she was a lonely one. At that time she did not know anyone to whom she felt she could confide without reserve about the deeper problems of her life. Helena Banks was by now a faithful friend, but obviously she did not have the authority of a minister. Then a providential opening occurred. Margery's parents realised how she was placed and they felt impelled to put her into touch with an 'elder' who would give her wise guidance when needed. This prompted them to write to a minister who for many years had been the leading Congregationalist preacher of his day, renowned in America as well as in England, Dr George Campbell Morgan. In London he was the star preacher at the vast Westminster Chapel in Buckingham Gate, the city's main stronghold of fundamentalist Congregationalism. There he regularly drew congregations of more than two thousand, and in the huge auditorium, which has been likened to Charing Cross Station, they listened spellbound while with missionary fervour, in his rich, clear voice, he interpreted the Bible, sentence by sentence, word by word.

The letter was a happy inspiration and Margery soon met the famous preacher, a towering figure, thin and gaunt with beautiful white hair. He was old enough to be her father and during the ensuing years an affectionate father-and-daughter friendship grew up which was an invaluable support to Margery and a joy to both of them.

Margery was in her thirty-fifth year when for the first time, in March 1932, she read a paper before the British Homoeopathic

Society. It was on the subject of asthma, and her opening words are notable for their tone of humility. What a contrast to her over-confidence a few years earlier when she had championed high potencies with such naïve enthusiasm! At first, she said, when she had been asked to read a paper to the Society, she had been very much inclined to refuse. 'However,' she went on, 'I was rather persuaded into it on the spur of the moment and afterwards was faced with the frightful problem of choosing a subject.' There did not seem to be anything she could possibly write about, she said, but on looking into her out-patient books and case notes she saw that asthma seemed to crop up again and again. She found that she had had at least sixty cases of asthma to tackle in her first five and a half years of general practice. Nevertheless she felt she had to apologise for her lack of experience.

In her lecture she explained that the cases she had found most difficult were those where there was a family history of asthma, because 'suggestibility or hysteria' was so often present. But, she said, she was quite convinced that these cases could be cured in spite of the neurotic element. She went on to tell how she had treated three members of an asthmatic family. The first of them who came to her was a woman of forty-three, Mrs B, small, very thin, nervous, inclined to get fits of depression about her health. For a year Margery did her best to 'work out' her case, trying various medicines in turn including *Arsenicum* and *Pulsatilla* (wind flower) – all to no avail. Then she decided to try *Kali sulphuricum* (potassium sulphate) in a high potency and this proved immediately right. Mrs B had been steadily better ever since, and latterly she had very seldom had a 'bad day', perhaps only once in two or three months.

The next member of the family to be treated was Mrs B's forty-one-year-old brother, Mr G, who had been suffering increasingly severe attacks of asthma for six years. He was a keen gardener, and the attacks were always worse at weekends after he had been working in the garden. 'I was tempted to

give him the *Kali sulph.* which had so helped his sister,'
Margery said. But when she studied the case in detail she
realised that it would not really 'fit'. Instead she gave him
Carbo veg., and for six months he was very much better, in
spite of continuing his weekend gardening. Then he had
another attack, and she gave him another dose of *Carbo veg.* A
year passed with no further trouble, and Margery had recently
heard from his sister that he considered his asthma was cured.

Mrs B's son was Margery's third patient in that family. He
was starting to be asthmatic, and had had two definite attacks
when she first saw him. The boy was scared and tongue-tied,
but she was able to learn enough to judge which medicine was
likely to help. She gave him *Natrum sulphuricum* (sodium
sulphate) in a high potency. That was two and a half years ago
and he had not had any hint of trouble since.

In the discussion that followed the lecture Margery was
warmly congratulated by her leading colleagues – all of them
men. Within the homoeopathic fraternity, at this stage of her
career, there seems to have been no whiff of prejudice against
her on grounds of sex. She was not in any way regarded as a
woman trespassing on male preserves. Dr Wheeler, who had
retired in 1928, but who still played an active part in the
Society, said he had listened to the paper with extraordinary
interest; he hoped that Dr Blackie would some time group her
sixty cases to show how the results worked out as a whole.
Margery's friend Frank Bodman, who although he was by
now practising in Bristol always came to London for the
Society's meetings, praised her paper and commented that
what had been particularly valuable was the wealth of clinical
observation recorded with regard to the medicines given, and
the fact that certain of them had failed. 'Dr Blackie had been
frank in stating when her prescriptions had gone wrong and
when they had worked.'

Others, too, spoke with enthusiasm, but surely the tribute
that must have meant most to Margery was from Dr Borland.
He went so far as to say that the results she had given were

'astonishing', and that 'they could easily beat anything he could do himself'.

The year 1932 was a milestone not only in Margery's career but in the history of homoeopathy in Britain. It was a year when, for a brief moment, it seemed that the long-standing prejudice of the medical establishment was going to be set aside. Some optimists even believed that ostracism and ridicule were things of the past. This euphoria did not last long, nevertheless several events which took place during this year were pointers towards a happier future.

In was in 1932 that Dr John Weir became Sir John Weir KCVO, and this honour was both a tribute to his attendance upon members of the royal family – he had been Physician-in-Ordinary to the Prince of Wales for nearly ten years – and also a sign of official recognition for homoeopathy itself. For although British royalty had relied upon homoeopathic remedies for generations, this was the first time that a homoeopath had been knighted.

Sir John was in touch with some of the leading figures in the medical world, including Lord Dawson, and he lost no time in making use of his new status. Plans were under way at the time to celebrate the centenary of the British Medical Association, and he suggested that homoeopathy might be included in the centenary proceedings 'if its case were cogently put'. As a result he was invited to speak at a special meeting of the Royal Society of Medicine, and his address, 'British Homoeopathy in the last hundred years', was subsequently published in the *British Medical Journal*. A further repercussion was that the libraries of the Royal Society of Medicine, the British Medical Association and the Royal College of Physicians agreed to accept collections of homoeopathic textbooks. This was not Sir John's only diplomatic coup in 1932. In the same year – so one of his admirers has put it – he 'invaded' the Royal Society of Medicine to read another paper, 'Homoeopathy, an Explanation of its Principles'.

All this leads one to ask, what sort of man was Sir John? What was his character, what were his main achievements? Furthermore how did he and his doings impinge upon Margery's life and work? Weir, like Borland, came from Glasgow, and he had the same qualities of kindliness, common sense, and dedication to his work. But in looks and character as well as manner the two were utterly different. Perhaps this is one of the reasons why Margery never got on well with Sir John.

In spite of many years of living in London, Weir never lost his Scottish accent. When he was knighted, at the age of fifty-three, he was still the well-to-do Scottish gentleman, clubman and golfer, a great teller of 'pawky jokes' and 'wee stories'. He was a thrifty Scot but in little ways he was generous; he often gave boxes of Lindt chocolate to his colleagues' wives. A diplomatist at heart, a confirmed bachelor, he was meticulously neat in his dress – and in his thinking. It is said that once, when he went to dinner at a friend's house, he got up between the courses to straighten a picture that was slightly askew.

As a homoeopath his greatest gift was undoubtedly in teaching. Margery herself, in *The Patient, Not the Cure*, paid tribute to this, and others who worked with him have acknowledged, almost with awe, his faithfulness as a teacher and as an upholder of the standards of homoeopathy. Appointed Compton Burnett Professor in 1911, he continued giving his regular lectures for as long as fifty years. These lectures took place within the British Homoeopathic Society, a body in which Weir played a vital part. Almost as soon as he joined the Society in 1909 he initiated changes that were much needed in its postgraduate teaching. In other words he laid the foundations upon which Margery, many years later, was destined to build.

Of his talents as a physician it has been said that 'no one had a better grasp of essentials or a quicker eye for detail, all controlled by strong Scottish common sense'. And he had a pleasantly informal idiom. He once said that if a patient seemed to be secretive he would explain that he was being given a jigsaw puzzle to solve, and he could not possibly do so if half a dozen pieces were hidden away. One of his younger colleagues has recalled that his ward rounds were always interesting: 'Although he was physician to the royal family . . . his kindness and skill were equally available to all the patients in the hospital.' And often his characteristic sense of humour came to the fore. 'On one occasion, after looking at an X-ray of the skull of a patient being investigated for headaches, Sir John turned to the patient (who was free from headache at the time) and said "We've done an X-ray of your head and I'm sorry to say we can't find anything in it".'

As regards Weir's standing among his fellow physicians, one of them wrote after his death, 'I will always picture him as the kindly father figure of the British homoeopaths.' But another, who perhaps knew him better, hinted that he was something of an autocrat. To the younger generation, he said, Sir John must sometimes have appeared an authority figure who got his way all too easily. A further reservation was expressed by a colleague who questioned whether he possessed the same deep knowledge of homoeopathy as Borland, Wheeler and Clarke. It was well known that Weir never hesitated to ask for a second opinion. Some would regard this as a matter for congratulation, and it may well have been an indication of personal humility – despite his many honours and high position he remained in some respects a humble man – but on the other hand it may have shown a fundamental diffidence due to a lack of understanding.

To return to the contrast between Sir John and Dr Borland, there was an occasion in the 1930s when Margery did not hide where her sympathies lay – an occasion that was to have far-reaching repercussions. It was a tradition that at the annual staff dinners of the London Homoeopathic Hospital the guests should themselves provide the entertainment, chiefly

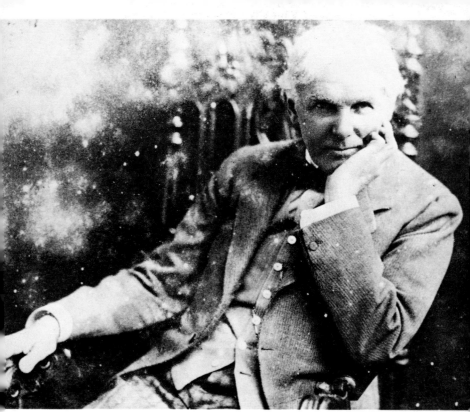

9 Dr John Henry Clarke

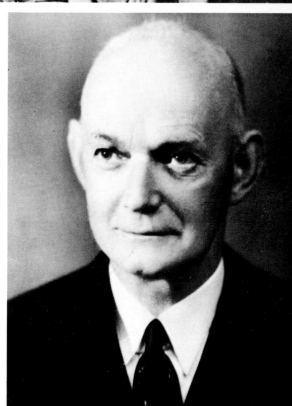

10 Dr Douglas Borland

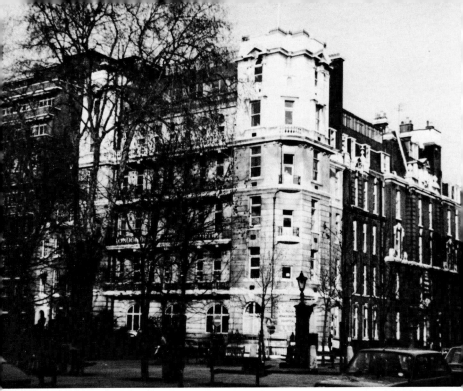

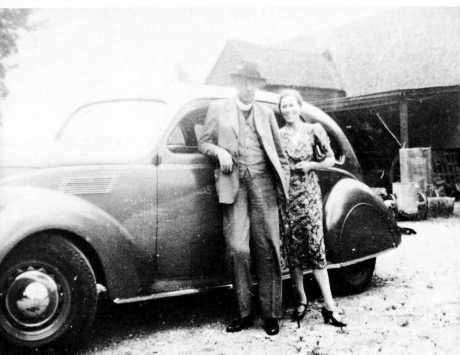

11 The Royal London Homoeopathic Hospital

12 Margery with Dr George Campbell Morgan

by means of doggerel verses lampooning well-known hospital personalities. At one of these dinners Margery contributed a composition of her own, 'The Cure of the Chronic Invalid (by himself)' which consisted of good-humoured caricatures of the hospital's leading physicians. It tells more of her feelings about Weir and Borland than any carefully worded obituaries or tributes.

> . . . For twenty-five or thirty years
> I suffered agony and tears . . .
> I placed myself in various hands . . .
> And found no remedy at all –
> My tottering hopes began to fall
> Until a friend I chanced to meet
> Said 'Why not try Great Ormond Street?'

> . . . The first Physician I met here
> Was called, I fancy, Dr Weir.
> A large man with a rosy face
> He talked at an alarming pace,
> Percussed my lungs, and banged my thighs
> And told me stories thick as flies.
> My heart went thump – my heart went hop,
> I thought that he would never stop.

> I came all over feeling queer
> And tottered out from Dr Weir
> Replete with anecdotes galore
> But as to my
> Pet maladie
> No wiser than I was before . . .

> And I was recommended then
> To Dr Borland – best of men.
> He sat me down upon a chair
> And stared with an absorbing stare.
> I felt his eyes investigate
> The deepest secrets of my state.
> I almost heard him count my sins –
> He knew them all, their outs and ins.

His stare bored down into my heart,
I felt the perspiration start –
My feet, my knees, my hands, my head,
All shook with a consuming dread.

I almost melted on the mat,
I simply rattled where I sat.
Oh! What a power for a Physician
To know by force of intuition
His patient's scandalous condition.

When I had almost ceased to hope
I thought I saw his fingers grope,
And from his pocket came to light
A tiny powder wrapped in white.
One sinewy arm he forward flung
And placed that powder on my tongue –
Scarce had I swallowed the contents
I felt its marvellous influence –
I ceased to sweat – I ceased to shake
I ceased to gibber and to quake
I felt as certain as old Nick
That Dr B had done the trick.

What an experience indeed
For one so long an invalid!

The laughter that greeted Margery's verses can well be imagined. But one person in her audience was not at all amused. Sir John never forgave her for making fun of him.

General Practitioner

From the very start of her practice Margery kept one morning a week for what she called her 'open consultations', mornings when anyone could come without an appointment. So she never knew whether there would be ten, twenty, or thirty names on her list. But however many came she always made a point of conducting each patient from the waiting room herself. This was not just a matter of courtesy. She had found that it was astonishing what one could learn about someone just by shaking hands and leading him or her into the consulting room. She even believed that the initial handshake was so vital that you could not make a complete diagnosis without it.

Hahnemann had once said that in taking a case the most important symptoms were the mental ones: 'It is the mental state which takes priority of consideration in the selection of the remedy.' So when Margery entered her waiting room, during the fleeting moments of the all-important face-to-face encounter, while she was giving a smiling welcome, she was simultaneously gaining an impression of the patient's 'mental state'. Demeanour, posture, facial expression, mannerisms, tone of voice, gestures; all of these counted for much. For, as Hahnemann taught, the aim of the homoeopath is to restore the patient to wholeness both of mind and body, and as Margery herself always maintained, her purpose was not to fight a disease as such, but to help the patient, by means of the right therapeutic stimuli, to overcome – unconsciously – his own unique reactions to stress, whether mental, emotional, physical, bacteriological, or just the everyday stresses and strains of life.

A vivid picture of Margery as a young general practitioner has been given by one of her patients who was a girl when her mother first took her to Alfred Place in June 1934. She subsequently returned often, and her memories are of special interest as showing how Margery appeared to a patient in the 1930s.

> Dr Blackie held surgeries on Mondays and Fridays (4 p.m. to 6 p.m.) and on Wednesdays (11 a.m. to 1 p.m.). My visits were mainly on a Monday when the waiting room would be filled with patients. Dr Blackie always came into the waiting room to fetch the next patient, calling some of them by their Christian names . . .
>
> She was quick in her diagnosis of what was wrong, asking very few questions . . . [and she] was always so very kind; I remember occasions when she put her arm about my shoulders in a sympathetic gesture . . . One came away feeling that one's symptoms had hardly been touched upon, and yet after a few doses of medicine the cure had begun.

Apparently in those days Margery, who had no head for money, ignored the usual formalities concerning fees:

> The fee was given to her personally; she would just thrust it into a pigeon-hole on her desk. I remember so often her saying 'Is that alright? Can you manage that?', or if for some reason or other one asked how much, the amount she mentioned was always lower than one would have expected.
>
> In my opinion Dr Blackie cared for every one of her patients, deciding what was best for each individually, giving advice when asked for, always with that same care and concern.

Although 'Dr Blackie was one of the kindest and most gentle of people' she could at times be quite stern, and this same patient remembers that as a teenager, and well into her twenties, she felt somewhat in awe of her.

For much of the week Margery devoted herself to her practice, absorbed in the problems of her private patients, who were of all ages and from all walks of life.* But she also took her responsibilities at the hospital very seriously, and in this, as in so much else, she shared the views of Dr Borland. He had once said, speaking of the role of a hospital physician, 'You are appointed to take on duties which are more or less honorary; but these duties are very much more serious and responsible than the duties of a medical man . . . Difficult cases are sent up to all the hospitals under the belief that the medical staff know a little more than their professional brethren outside.'

During most of the 1930s, at the hospital, Margery continued as an assistant physician in the childrens' department, and at the nurses' home nearby. But Margery's own home in Tuesdays and Fridays. For some time already she had been accustomed to out-patient work, because another of the hospital's physicians, Dr Margaret Tyler (daughter of Sir Henry Tyler, a great benefactor of homoeopathy) had for many years been running an out-patient clinic for mentally handicapped children, and Margery had been allowed to help her.

In her time Dr Tyler was a dominant figure at the hospital, and indeed in the whole homoeopathic scene. Both as a teacher with sound academic knowledge and as an author with a breezy freshness of style her influence was enduring. At the hospital, which she had served with single-minded dedication since the beginning of the First World War, she was the first woman homoeopath to attain senior status, and if Sir John Weir was the hospital's father figure, its mother figure was Margaret Tyler. Margery herself described her (in her provocative after-dinner 'poem') as 'a stately dame', with 'an air of common sense, mixed with profound benevolence'.

There seems little doubt that as a personality the 'stately

* It seems that she also sometimes prescribed 'on the side'. There is a story that in the 1930s she knew an amateur homoeopath who worked in the Covent Garden market. He would phone her up and say 'I've got a couple of cases', and next morning she would be off to Covent Garden at 4.30 a.m. to advise.

dame' was not especially congenial to Margery, perhaps because she was a devoted friend and admirer of Sir John Weir. Yet some of her most strongly held views coincide with those later held by Margery herself, and it is noteworthy that the two women worked regularly together at a time when Margery was accumulating experience. Dr Tyler was a great believer in going to 'the fountainhead', as she termed Hahnemann, and she feared that much contemporary homoeopathic practice was diverging from the 'classical' ideal. She was deeply concerned, too, for the future supply of homoeopathic physicians, as in those days there was no provision for co-ordinated postgraduate training, or for the acquiring of official qualifications.

Margery's clinical experience with Dr Tyler was the basis of the second paper she read to the British Homoeopathic Society, in 1934. Entitled 'The Clinical Aspect of the Backward Child', it gives a good idea of the scope of their work together, for a succession of case histories are grouped under four headings: congenital cases, cases due to birth injuries, endocrine abnormalities, and 'induced backwardness'. Margery's general tone shows that she was gradually gathering confidence, though she was still very conscious of being a beginner. After describing one case, which was currently under treatment, she confessed disarmingly, 'I'm frankly puzzled as to what to do next. I should very much like to hear the opinion of the meeting.'

But some of the cases she described were impressive success stories. Under the heading 'birth injuries' she told about a boy who was brought to the out-patient department at the age of two, unable to walk or stand and acutely nervous. His mother gave a history of having had 'a seventy-two hours confinement and instruments'. During the ensuing few months Margery tried giving him various different medicines, chiefly *Natrum muriaticum* (sodium chloride) and *Borax* (borate of sodium) in a very high potency, and by his third birthday he was talking pretty well. After a year of treatment he was walking perfectly and was entirely changed in appearance. Another little boy suffering from birth injuries appeared to be a hopeless imbecile when she first saw him, and she thought he would never be able to walk alone. This time she found that *Baryta carbonica* (carbonate of barium) was what helped him most. After a year and a half of homoeopathic treatment he was on his feet and trying to form words and talk.

Finally she dealt with cases of 'induced backwardness', a term which she realised needed explanation.

> I consider that every normal child has an expectation of success or failure in every subject he tackles, or skill he seeks to attain. This expectation is usually exerted quite unconsciously, and only if the child is thwarted or pampered unnecessarily will his expectation develop along the lines of failure, and then, although he may be really normal mentally he will become stupid and seemingly below the average in intelligence.

She had found this sort of trouble very common. In such cases, where children were called stupid, peculiar or backward, great benefit had often been derived from homoeopathic remedies.

For instance there was a boy called Peter, who was ten when she first saw him. He was the only child of definitely nervy parents. The headmaster of his preparatory school had written home to say that his nerves were dreadful. He was terrified by any sudden noise and could not stand still for two minutes. In front of strangers he had developed a stutter, and he constantly played up to his reputation of being peculiar. He arrived home for the holidays inclined to burst into tears at the slightest provocation and he was exceedingly argumentative, with the terms 'peculiar', 'odd', 'backward' running through his mind.

Margery at first gave him *Argentum nitricum* (silver nitrate) but he did not do well on it. She then tried a series of other medicines, and finally found the right one. *Thuja occidentalis* (derived from the African evergreen 'tree of life') brought about an astonishing improvement in him.

He is now fourteen and getting on well. He has caught up in his school work in the subjects in which he was so lamentably stupid, and in many other subjects he is exceptionally sharp. He still finds difficulty in facing noise but that is becoming less and less marked . . . He is just going on to a Public School where I think he will take his place normally with the other boys.

During her early years as a doctor Margery was not only accumulating knowledge of children's diseases. It is true that her main responsibilities in the hospital had been, and still were, concerned with prescribing for children of all ages, children suffering from every kind of disease and complaint. But at the same time, in her practice, many of her patients – in fact the majority – were adults, and her third paper for the British Homoeopathic Society was on the subject of rheumatoid arthritis. This was a disease, she said, that she had treated very often and which she had *enjoyed* treating. 'I can never see a case of rheumatoid arthritis, however bad it may be,' she said, 'without feeling that a great deal ought to be possible towards curing the patient with homoeopathic remedies . . . How frequently I have failed I am not stopping to relate, but with different methods and widely different remedies I have obtained some interesting results.'

For the arthritic she nearly always prescribed high potencies. She had found that this kind of 'shock treatment' was usually needed. Results were often 'miraculous', though at the start it sometimes took a period of experimentation to identify the right remedy, or series of remedies, for a particular person. This had been so in the case of one of the patients she had watched over, a middle-aged workman, a navvy in the building trade. He had been off work, with no use in his arms, and tormented by pain in neck, arms and back, for fourteen months when she first saw him – a thin miserable-looking little man, with a gray face and drawn expression, who suffered from frightful nightmares. She had begun by trying in turn *Rhus tox.*, *Silica* and other medicines, but to no avail. Then she gave him *Causticum* (hydrated lime) and this brought the first sign of improvement, with a lessening of the pain in his back. 'This man has gone on steadily improving ever since,' she said, 'mostly on *Causticum*, but *Natrum carbonicum* (sodium carbonate), *Sulphur*, and *Kali bichromicum* (bichromate of potash) have all helped to clear up some phase of his trouble.' After a year he had almost entirely recovered. 'He is now doing a builder's work as usual,' she reported, 'and wielding a fourteen-pound hammer for several hours each day. He still has slight stiffness in the hands and feet, although he can move and grasp properly.' She added however that the symptom she had not yet been able to relieve was his tendency to bad dreams. 'They are still terribly vivid . . . and I should be most grateful for suggestions as to what will help that.'

The years just before the Second World War were years when homoeopaths in Britain were devoting much thought to rheumatic diseases, and in 1938 the Congress of the British Homoeopathic Society took as its subject 'The Rheumatisms'. By this time Margery was not only a Fellow of the Society but a member of its Council, and when plans were being made for the congress her name was one of the five put forward to represent London – second only on the list to Sir John Weir.

During her years as a doctor she had had much experience of dealing with 'ordinary rheumatism' as well as arthritis, and she admitted that she found it much more difficult to treat. On the whole it responded best to low potencies, but she found that the 'right' medicine could be 'exasperatingly elusive'. The only path was to keep on trying different remedies.

One of her cases of rheumatism that had illustrated this is of special interest as an example of what homoeopaths call 'constitutional prescribing'. (If a particular medicine can be correctly judged to match the temperament and physiology of a particular person, it is known as that person's 'constitutional drug', and it can stimulate a vital healing reaction which often resolves a recurrent problem.) The case concerned a middle-aged woman who had developed sudden acute rheumatism in the right shoulder after a very damp spell of weather. Within a few weeks it got so bad that she could not raise her arm, do her hair, or put on a coat without help. Margery gave her *Rhus tox.*, but this had very little effect. She tried the additional aid of massage and radiant heat but still with no result. Then by chance the patient gave her a crucial clue; she mentioned that sea air made her feel temporarily worse, also that she preferred salt with her food to any other seasoning. Thereupon Margery gave her a dose of *Natrum muriaticum* in a high potency. The rheumatism cleared up immediately and did not return. 'In this case', so Margery later wrote, 'I think I prescribed entirely locally in the first instance, and that *Nat. mur.* was the patient's constitutional drug and therefore cleared the condition at once.'

The war years brought major changes for Margery, not only in her professional work. She was by now in her early forties, and her private life was assuming a new pattern. Her parents' home in Norfolk had hitherto linked her firmly to her family, although she had not often been able to visit Downham Market. But after her father died in 1936 the Norfolk ménage came to an end, and a few years later, in 1941, her mother also died. And although two of her sisters, Kay and Lillian (Mrs Townend) were working in London, their paths did not often cross with hers.

But beyond her own family circle warm friendships were not lacking. There was her day-to-day companionship with Helena Banks, who was becoming more and more indispensable as her partner at Thurloe Street. And off-duty the two shared an absorbing interest, an enthusiasm for birdwatching. Helena had a cottage at East Dean on the Sussex coast, and after a break there with Margery she would eagerly tell her patients that they had been seeing long-tailed tits, or kestrels or spotted woodpeckers.

Equally vital to Margery, at this time, in quite a different way, was her relationship with Dr Campbell Morgan, which had blossomed into a very close friendship with his family as well as himself. During the 1930s 'Blackie', as Dr Morgan and his wife always called her, accompanied them on several holidays. Margery was a good driver – at this time she had a Buick – and she enjoyed acting as chauffeuse.

But there was much more to their friendship than holiday outings. Just before the war, and on through the war years, Margery was constantly in attendance on Dr Morgan and his wife. His daughter Ruth (Mrs Shute) recalls that Blackie used to come almost every morning to the Campbell Morgan flat at the St Ermin's Hotel in Westminster, to see how they were and whether they needed anything. Especially after Ruth's marriage in 1941 Margery often took them shopping and helped generally, this in spite of her usual heavy burden of work – the hospital, the practice, and the home visiting which she regarded as all-important.

Margery's daughterly devotion to the great preacher was a top priority in her life. And meantime, on the spiritual level, she had come to rely more and more upon the inspiration of Dr Morgan's teachings. She went regularly to hear him on Sundays, and also – until the air-raids began – she attended his 'Friday evenings' when with a blackboard in the imposing mahogany pulpit at the Westminster Chapel he used to give 'Bible lessons', expounding the scriptures in his compelling style to the crowds who came from all over London, drawn by his magnetic personality. The intimate dependence on the Bible for ethical guidance which so characterised Margery's thinking in later life undoubtedly gathered strength at this time.

A further bond between Margery and Dr Morgan was that he and his family were firm believers in homoeopathy. Not long after she met him he became her patient, and his gratitude for her ministrations was profound, as witnessed by the dedication of his book *The Parables and Metaphors of Our Lord*, one of his many biblical commentaries, which was published in 1943. It is dedicated to 'My friend and physician, Margery G. Blackie, M.D., to whose skill and devotion I owe more than I can tell'.

In the light of all this, we can well imagine what a desolation of grief Margery must have suffered when Dr Morgan, in his eighty-third year, died in May 1945. Thus ended a chapter in her emotional life. A terrible gap was left – but not for very long.

During Dr Morgan's latter years at the Westminster Chapel his responsibilities had been shared with a younger minister, Dr Martyn Lloyd-Jones, then in his early forties. Dr Lloyd-Jones had earlier trained in medicine, and as a brilliant young doctor at Bart's had worked under Lord Horder. But his vocation to the ministry became so compelling that at the age of twenty-seven he abandoned the medical profession, turning his back on what promised to be a highly successful career.

Like Dr Morgan he was a preacher who attracted enormous congregations – people of all ages, nationalities, denominations, levels of society – but in manner and in looks they were entirely different. Dr Lloyd-Jones, dark and good-looking, appeared much more like a doctor in his consulting room than a minister in his chapel. When he preached he was serious and unsmiling although out of the pulpit he was warmly genial. As to his style, he did not use the language of the professional evangelist. He had a clear and analytical mind and at the same time the ability to think and speak on spiritual matters in an everyday idiom, though he was not in the least chatty. He spoke with passionate conviction and deep concern, and this had a powerful appeal.

When Margery first knew him, and listened to his sermons, she did not take kindly to him, for his whole personality was so different from that of her beloved Dr Morgan. She was even somewhat prejudiced against him, for she felt he had not co-operated with Dr Morgan as he should have. But in due course, as the years passed after the older man's death, she was able to find in him a wise counsellor and an understanding friend. She also came to have affectionate respect for his beautiful wife, Bethan, who like her husband had formerly been a doctor, and through these friendships she kept up her links with the Westminster Chapel; she also became a member of the Christian Medical Fellowship.

Margery's professional life, on the everyday level, was not so much disrupted by the war as one might have expected. Although many people had left London she was busier than ever, since quite a few homoeopathic doctors joined the Services. For a time she saw patients at 148 Harley Street as well as at her home, and in her hospital work, too, she had a heavy load, for in 1939 she had been appointed physician in charge of out-patients.

During the Blitz, bombs fell on Great Ormond Street, causing much havoc at the London Homoeopathic Hospital and at the nurses' home nearby. But Margery's own home in Kensington was not hit (incidentally, Alfred Place had by now been renamed, so the house had become number 18 Thurloe Street) and from September 1943 it was possible to establish the practice there on a more permanent basis; thanks to a financial outlay on the part of Helena Banks the freehold was purchased.

Despite the raids and all the disruptions of war, the British Homoeopathic Society continued to function, and the Society's journal was still published though on a reduced scale. Sir John Weir, Dr Borland and Dr Wheeler still gave their lectures and tutorials in the hospital, and meetings of the Society were also held occasionally. For example in December 1940 there was a discussion, led by Dr Borland, on air-raid casualties and how best to use homoeopathic remedies to help the injured and those whose nerves had been shattered. This was a subject on which Margery herself later spoke. During the raids, she said, most people were able to control their emotion and show no fear. But when control gave way, homoeopathic first aid was able to help very greatly. 'There was the woman having hysterics – sobbing uncontrollably – who only stopped to take long sighing breaths. People tried to comfort her, but it had no effect. She wouldn't listen. *Ignatia* (St

Ignatius bean) helped her to control herself very quickly.'
Then there were the people who, in spite of great fear, were
able to endure the first few raids. As each day passed, the dread
of the night made them increasingly terrified. They became
more fidgety and unable to compose themselves until they
could bear it no longer and took flight to the country. 'If they
were given *Argentum nit.* they were able to carry on again, and
they soon learned that a further dose would stop that terror of
anticipation whenever it began to come back.' Others dreaded
the nightly raids so much, she said, that they constantly had to
be given *Phosphoricum acidum* (phosphoric acid) to prevent the
diarrhoea of anticipation.

Within the Society it was a time when there was a growing
awareness of new possibilities, and also a new interest in
developments that were taking place in other branches of
medicine. One sign of this was that the Society's journal now
included a section headed 'Critical digests from medical literature', with quotations from the *Lancet*, the *British Medical
Journal* etc. on such matters as the effects of penicillin and other
new drugs. Furthermore certain of the lectures that were now
read before the Society dealt with themes that opened strange
new vistas for the followers of Hahnemann.

Just before the war, for instance, in February 1939, a lecture
was given by a homoeopath called Dr James Turner entitled
'Rudolf Steiner – A fresh outlook on the Etiology★ of Disease'. This was the first time that a summary of Steiner's
philosophy of medicine had been presented to the Society. Dr
Turner explained that Steiner's views on the causes of disease
stemmed from his belief in a metaphysical aspect of physiology. 'Behind the material world which we can see, feel, hear,
smell and taste, there is an invisible supersensible world which
is visible to the clairvoyant.' According to Steiner, so Turner
claimed, most disease is caused by an imbalance between the
metaphysical 'force systems' such as the 'Etheric Body' and
the 'Astral Body', upon which the well-being of the person

★ The science, doctrine, or demonstration of causes.

depends. He ended his lecture with the following unequivocal assertion: 'It will be seen that the question of health or disease is based upon the relationship between the forces or activities of the physical substance of the body and of the various invisible bodies with which it is permeated.'

During the discussion that followed, one of the hospital's senior physicians, Dr William Ritchie McCrae, well known for his independent views, said that Steiner had many followers, and as physicians it was for them to know something about things outside their ken, so that when they met them in practice they would not be ignorant. Favourable comments were also made by several others, who thought that Steiner's theories might help to explain how high potencies worked. But one or two spoke more guardedly, admitting that they were out of their depth and showing clearly that they thought the whole subject was 'up in the clouds'.

In the clinical field, too, during the war years, there were changes. For example an innovation of a practical kind – an 'electro-medical' method of homoeopathic diagnosis – which was being developed in Glasgow by a Scottish homoeopath, the late Dr William Boyd, was gradually coming to be accepted by some of the physicians at the London hospital. Dr Boyd had found that by making use of a machine of his own invention which he called the Emanometer, in conjunction with specimens such as hair or blood, a patient's 'emanations' could be analysed and recorded (to emanate means 'to issue forth from a source, as fragrance emanates from flowers') and these emanations could then be matched up with potentially suitable homoeopathic remedies, with the aim of identifying the one which was ideal for this particular case.

Margery did not regard Boyd's method as in any way obviating the need for normal diagnostic practice, but she found it could provide a valuable short cut in certain difficult cases, and in June 1941 she read a short paper to the British Homoeopathic Society entitled 'Helps from the Emanometer'. She said that she often turned for help to Dr Boyd in cases where she had tried out all the obvious remedies without success, and in emergency cases where there was no time to try one remedy after another. She also stressed that when she sent him the patient's specimens, she also sent very full details of the symptoms. 'For a good many years now,' she asserted, 'I have appealed to Dr Boyd at least once a month for help in cases in which I have been badly stuck; and I have derived very great value from his work . . . He will do nothing unless he has received a full medical history, and as many homoeopathic symptoms as possible before making the tests.' 'So much so,' she went on, 'that on one occasion when I had omitted some important detail from my letter, I sent what I intended to be a night telegram with the missing symptoms, to be delivered with the letters next morning. Apparently this is not the way things are done in Scotland, for I learned later from Dr Boyd that he was awakened at 2 a.m. by resounding knocking at his door, and when he opened it a huge Post Office van, looking in the dark rather like an ambulance, was standing there. At his appearance the doors of the van were flung open and my telegram was produced. Since then I have been more careful about wiring.'

For homoeopathy in Britain the greatest change of all during the course of the war came about in the context of the revolution in the whole medical scene. Before the war actually began, the Emergency Medical Service, which had been formed under the Ministry of Health to deal with military and civilian casualties, had brought to light many inadequacies in the country's hospitals. The position of the voluntary hospitals was called in question, and for homoeopathy this was an alarming danger signal. Then at the end of 1942 came the Beveridge Report recommending the creation of a comprehensive health service.

Grave concern was felt in the homoeopathic fraternity, and it was realised that drastic moves were called for on the part of the British Homoeopathic Society if the status of its speciality

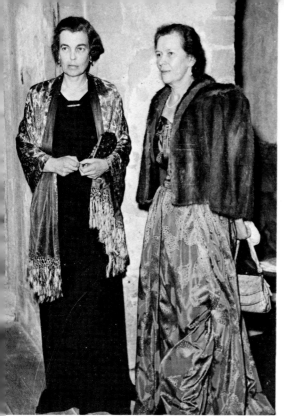

13 Musette Majendie (*l*)
with Margery

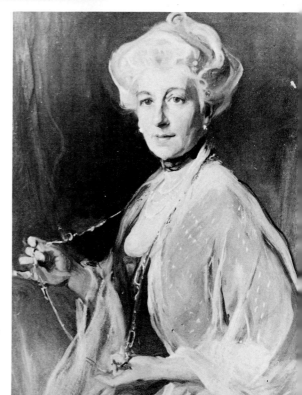

14 Lady Jane Lindsay

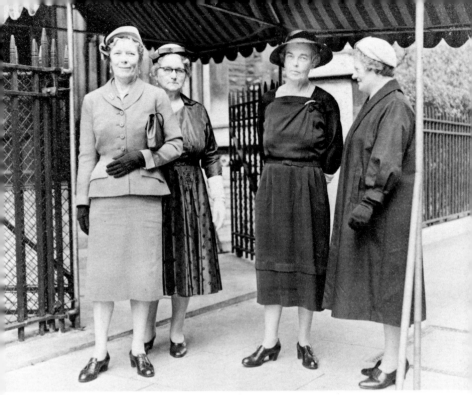

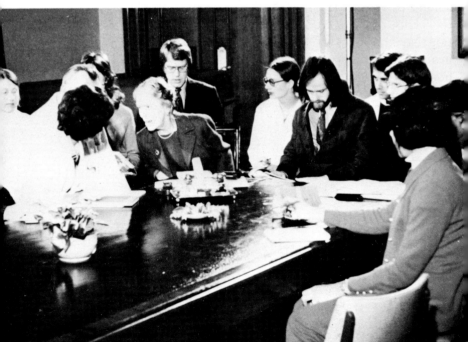

15 Going to a party: *l–r* Margery, Helena Banks,
Musette Majendie, Agnes Joyce

16 Margery and postgraduate students

was to be upheld in any post-war medical schemes. By this time Margery was one of the council's vice-presidents, so she was doubtless closely involved. A reorganisation of the whole medical profession was regarded as inevitable, though it seemed possible that there might be provision in certain hospitals for homoeopathic practitioners. In the anticipated new set-up, however, this would mean that anyone who applied for such a post would have to show some special qualification.

To meet this need the Society resolved to seek legal incorporation, by means of which it would be reconstituted as the British Faculty of Homoeopathy, with power to grant a diploma in homoeopathic medicine. This change of status – a 'protective act' rather than evidence of a change of heart in general attitude – was given royal approval by King George VI, and on 21 January 1944 the British Faculty of Homoeopathy came into being, replacing the British Homoeopathic Society which had been founded by Quin just a hundred years before. Thereafter its members had the right to inscribe the letters 'MF Hom.' after their names (a suggestion that the letters 'MFH' should be used had been rejected on grounds that they might be taken to mean 'Master of Foxhounds').

Sir John Weir was the first President of the Faculty as well as President of its research committee; Dr Borland was the education committee's chairman. At this initial stage Margery was not one of the Faculty's officers, but her time was soon to come.

PART TWO

Leading

Madam President

Margery's leadership in the world of British homoeopathy began all at once in 1949 with a leap to the top of the tree. She had already served an apprenticeship, as one of the vice-presidents of the British Homoeopathic Society, and now, in the newly formed Faculty, she was elected President. It is said that Sir John Weir did not favour the appointment but evidently he had to give way, and Margery's success in the presidential role is clear from the fact that, although the term of tenure is for one year, she was twice re-elected, in 1950 and again in 1951. She was the first woman ever to hold this position, and it is notable, too, that except for herself *all* the office-holders in the Faculty at this time – every one of them – were men; not only the vice-presidents, the treasurer and the nine council members, but also the many lesser officials such as the editor of the journal and members of the educational and research committees.

Thus her appointment was a resounding tribute, not only to her capabilities as a physician, but to herself as a person, to her dynamic character, her understanding of politics in the medical world, her ability to achieve, and to inspire others to achieve. In the light of all this, the fact that she was a woman was of minor importance.

Margery was now in her early fifties, and although at the hospital she was still only an assistant physician, she had, over twenty years of general practice, established a reputation for hard-working dedication and a flair for diagnosis, as well as for her remarkable successes in treating chronic diseases and ailments. But she had not hitherto made a mark in the homoeopathic world as a whole. In her lectures to the British Homoeopathic Society she had shown an apologetic shyness, and she very seldom took part in the discussions. Now however, in the presidential chair, her diffidence dropped away, giving place to a confident, almost aggressive frankness. Even when she opened her first presidential address she showed this new assurance, for she began by admitting that ever since she had been a student twenty-seven years before, when she had viewed the presidential chair with 'awe and admiration', it had been her one desire to sit in it herself. 'And here I am!' she exclaimed.

The keynote of her address, 'The Place of Homoeopathy in Modern Medicine', was optimistic enthusiasm. 'The homoeopath is no longer an outcast,' she declared, 'if not actually welcomed, he is at least admitted to the profession (here she referred to the acceptance of homoeopathy within the National Health Service). She went on to speak of some of the new applications of homoeopathic therapy in various fields – immunisation, pre-operative prophylaxis, burns, bacterial infection. Also the treatment of fractures. Homoeopathy was a blessing to the surgeon in the realm of fractures, she asserted. When treated with *Calcarea phosphorica* (phosphate of lime) and *Symphytum* (comfrey) fractures unite more quickly than those without. She herself had treated six old ladies over eighty with broken legs. None of them had had morphia or needed it (on account of having been given *Arnica*). All six recovered and were able to walk again as well as ever. Another old lady of ninety-six had fallen off a stool and cracked her pelvis. The skill of the surgeon plus homoeopathy had got her well in record time. 'And now,' Margery reported triumphantly, 'at ninety-eight, she is able to walk up and down stairs. Can any system except homoeopathy claim a hundred per cent recovery after fractured legs in patients over eighty?'

Finally she ended her address with a stirring outburst:

What, after all this, is the place of homoeopathy in modern medicine? I have tried to show that it is a system . . . practised by men and women within the body of the medical profession, who, availing themselves of all the modern methods of treatment, still find that with homoeopathic medicine they get results that thrill and amaze them and that would be deemed impossible by those of the orthodox school . . .

Perhaps we do not always realise to the full the greatness of our heritage. Our responsibility for its pure and truthful presentation is great indeed.

During Margery's first year as President she not only took the lead among her British colleagues, but also acted as hostess at an international gathering attended by delegates from all over the world. In July 1950 the Council of the International Homoeopathic League joined the Faculty of Homoeopathy and the British Homoeopathic Congress for a three-day conference in London. For the first time Margery was plunged into an international milieu, and she made many friends from abroad. Leading homoeopaths had come to the conference from near and far, and they brought with them news of developments in many countries: France, Germany, Holland, Italy, Switzerland, Argentina, Brazil, India, Mexico, Pakistan.

In an opening speech Margery spoke of the situation in Britain, in terms of optimism tempered by realism. 'The spread of homoeopathy has always been difficult,' she said. 'In the old days it was largely due to the prejudice and active antagonism of the medical profession as a whole. This grows less and less. Today the main obstacle is modern medicine with its dramatic results obtained by the recently discovered drugs, the sulphonamides, penicillin, streptomycin etc. Medicals find it difficult to believe that we have a better method and equally dramatic and very often more lasting results. However, we have more entries next year for our post-graduate course than ever before, and more patients demanding homoeopathy.'

Replying to Margery the President of the International Homoeopathic League, Dr Léon Renard of Paris, paid her a gallant tribute: 'I respectfully thank Dr Margery Blackie for her welcome . . . I know the impulse she is giving to the Faculty.' Then he went on to make a statement which may have caused some secret amusement to her male colleagues: 'She is the right man in the right place.'

In France, the conference was told, there was 'a daily increase of physicians . . . who practise homoeopathy and numerous students who seek instruction'. But full official recognition had not yet been gained. From Holland the news was less encouraging. Homoeopathy was being practised 'under great difficulties', and although there was a hospital near Utrecht, official recognition was withheld. The situation in Switzerland was rather more promising; there, despite a similar lack of official recognition, homoeopathy was receiving a 'sympathetic hearing from the general body of the medical profession'. Further organisation was needed but increased numbers were attending the twice-yearly reunions and in Basle there was a homoeopathic hospital. An active revival had gradually been taking place in Germany since the war, and a number of societies had been formed, with Frankfurt becoming the main centre for homoeopathic studies. News from Italy was of centres in Rome, Naples and Florence, and of a modern clinic in Rome where lecture courses were held; also a postgraduate two-year course 'with strict adherence to Hahnemannian classical homoeopathy'.

From further afield, an Argentinian doctor brought a glowing report of the situation in his country, where homoeopathy was 'gaining in prestige every day among all social classes'. About twenty-five years ago there had been only two or three homoeopathic doctors in Buenos Aires, and only one chemist where homoeopathic medicines could be obtained. Today, he said, there were more than two hundred doctors and 'four very important chemists'; one of these alone had an average output of ten thousand prescriptions a month. In Brazil, as in

Argentina, though more recently, there had been a surge of interest, with much publicity by means of the media. Official recognition had been granted, and homoeopathy was to be taught in all the medical schools.

Two additional reports, of exceptional interest, were from India and Pakistan. They brought out vividly how far the status of homoeopathy in those countries differs from its status in the West. In India, the conference was told, homoeopathy is not only recognised and aided by the Government (side by side with modern medicine) but in its basic principles and simplest forms it has been believed in and adhered to by the people for centuries, indeed from time immemorial. The cheap prices now of homoeopathic remedies brought them within reach of the rural population, and every village had its lay practitioner of homoeopathy, whose role was not unlike that of witch-doctor. The statistics were staggering to Western ears: the total number of so-called 'practising homoeopaths' in India was estimated at nearly a hundred thousand, and of these some seventy-five thousand were laymen – self-taught, and lacking in formal qualifications, but nevertheless 'doing wonderful service to the poor suffering millions of India'. It was being realised increasingly, however, that India was in acute need of *qualified* homoeopaths, trained in the classical homoeopathy of Hahnemann, and a few specialist colleges already existed. But only a small proportion of practitioners had attended them, and even fewer had taken preliminary courses in general medicine; such courses were usually regarded as too time-consuming and not strictly necessary, when the need to replace the entirely unqualified lay practitioners was so urgent. A move was afoot to establish at least one government-financed homoeopathic college in each of the state capitals, with diploma courses of four or five years, and a 'model syllabus' had been drafted.

The report from Pakistan showed that there too homoeopathy was very popular with the people. Practitioners numbered about three thousand, and eight hundred dispensaries were in action. During the three years since the Republic of Pakistan had come into being several homoeopathic societies had been formed, and a further piece of news – a fascinating detail – was that Hahnemann's birthday on 10 April was celebrated each year all over the country.

On the third day of the London conference the Duke of Gloucester, accompanied by the Duchess, brought a message of good wishes from King George VI. For the royal family's association with homoeopathy had not been endangered by the establishment of the National Health Service in 1948; in fact it had been emphasised. In the very same year the London Homoeopathic Hospital had been empowered to add the word 'Royal' to its name.

Before the congress ended, a group photograph of the crowd of delegates was taken outside the hospital, in Queen Square. Sitting at the centre, side by side, were Margery and Sir John Weir. What a contrast! Weir was then in his eighties, a stout ponderous figure, with sparse white hair and a heavy drooping moustache – the grand old man of British homoeopathy. Beside him sat Margery, slim, erect, her poise almost regal, and with a look of gracious happiness on her face. She looked elegant, too, wearing a neat dark frock, with discreet touches of jewellery and a little halo hat framing her face.

Margery's first year as 'Madam President' was a milestone in her career. At the end of it, at a Faculty meeting, even Sir John Weir himself voiced a warm tribute: 'I think we ought to propose a vote of thanks to the President. I want to congratulate her on having survived the notoriety of being the first woman president, and secondly – if she does not think it presumptuous – I want to congratulate her on the way in which she has performed her duties.'

Margery very seldom allowed herself any breaks from her intensive professional routine, but at about this time she did have a few weeks' respite; she went on a cruise to Madeira. So far as we know it was an uneventful cruise. But during the course of it an incident occurred which remained long in her memory. This incident concerned an intensely controversial matter which was, and is, a perennial problem for homoeopaths, namely the rooted prejudice against homoeopathy felt by many members of the medical establishment.

'Years ago on a cruise to Madeira,' Margery later recalled, 'the purser, at whose table I was sitting, developed a facial paralysis and disappeared. A famous neurologist whom I knew was a passenger and had been asked to see him. He told me that it was such a pity there was nothing they could do for him till he got back to England – three weeks ahead – when he could have electric treatment. I said "A little homoeopathic *Causticum* would help." "What a pity we haven't got any", said he with a smile. "But I have", I replied, "I always carry a case of medicines with me." Never was there such a change. From being a friendly colleague he became an expressionless bit of granite and started talking about the weather.'

This little anecdote shows that Margery's claim in her first presidential speech, the claim that the antagonism of the medical profession was growing less and less, was certainly optimistic. It also raises the question, *what is the reason for the 'rooted prejudice'?* There are, in fact, several reasons for it. The antagonism can be attributed to four main causes: ignorance, misconceptions, the activities of unqualified homoeopaths, and the lack of a scientific explanation of how homoeopathy works.

Ignorance of homoeopathy among doctors results primarily from the pressures of medical life. There is no time to look into the matter objectively, so it is assumed from hearsay that homoeopathy is some sort of faith-healing based on old wives' tales. As to the more realistic misconceptions, one of the commonest is the idea that homoeopathy is the same thing as herbalism. Few are aware that many homoeopathic remedies are prepared from natural sources other than plants; for example from metallic materials such as silver, copper and lead – these are ground up with lactose (sugar of milk) so as to be

soluble for dilution; also from non-metallic elements such as
sulphur and tellurium; also from pathological tissues com-
parable to vaccines; also from animal secretions – bee stings,
the poison of certain spiders, and most notably from snake
venom. The important homoeopathic medicine *Lachesis* is
derived from the venom of the bushmaster snake.★

Besides all this, the irresponsible activities of unqualified
enthusiasts (and there are great numbers of them) have caused
many doctors to condemn all homoeopaths as quacks. It is not
widely known that to be a qualified homoeopath in Britain
means that you have already been fully trained in general
medicine.

But in recent times the main reason for the 'rooted prejudice' – such as that which Margery encountered on the
Madeira cruise – has been the lack of any full scientific
explanation as to how homoeopathy works, or, to be more
precise, how the dynamic action of homoeopathic remedies,
with their infinitesimal doses of potentised medicines, can be
defined and measured. During the early years of her practice,
Margery's main knowledge of this field came from the researches of the brilliant Scottish homoeopath, Dr William
Boyd, whose invention the Emanometer had, as we know,
often helped her to find appropriate remedies in difficult cases.
In Glasgow, in the Boyd Medical Research Trust laboratories,
further experimental work in electro-physics was continuing,
in an attempt to discover what form of energy was involved in
the action of homoeopathic potencies, and to explore the

★ The story of how *Lachesis* came to be a homoeopathic medicine was often
related by Margery. The first 'proving' was carried out – or rather under-
gone – in the early nineteenth century by Hahnemann's disciple, Dr
Constantine Hering. While in Dutch Guiana, with his wife, collecting
botanical specimens, the native Indians told him so much about the powerful venom of the Surukuku snake, that he offered a reward for a live
specimen. When they succeeded in capturing one he carefully held its head
and 'milked' the venom onto granules of sugar of milk. The mere handling
of the poison threw him into a high fever 'with delirium and mania', but after
a time he fell asleep. On waking he immediately questioned his wife: 'What
did I do? What did I say?', and the symptoms were recorded in detail.

interaction of potentised medicines and the bio-physical properties of the human body.

Funds were urgently needed to support this research and Margery had been involved for the first time in fund-raising in the spring of 1947, when a function was staged at the Chelsea Town Hall. On 21 May her devoted friend Dame Myra Hess whom she often helped with homoeopathic prescriptions* had given a piano recital there in aid of the Boyd Trust. Princess Alice, Duchess of Gloucester, already for some years an enthusiastic supporter of homoeopathy, attended the recital, and it is notable that this was the first time – the first of many times – when such an occasion organised by Margery had royal support.

* Margery later told of an occasion when Dame Myra was attacked by severe back pain. She was X-rayed and early arthritis was distinctly shown in her lower back. If her back was pressed in any way she felt pain going up to her head, and then all over her, so that she could hardly go on. She had to push herself up from the piano-stool after playing. The homoeopathic remedy *Tellurium* cured her, and her X-ray plates confirmed this, to the amazement of those who had seen her in the early stages.

A New Life

New personal relationships came to Margery after the end of the war which were soon to transform her way of life. Indeed, in the perspective of her life as a whole one can truly say that it consisted of two parts, the years before 1945 and those that followed. After 1945 the whole rhythm of her existence took a new shape, although her work as a dedicated homoeopath continued as before, or rather it continued with a new intensity, as she undertook additional responsibilities.

By the time the war ended, her private practice was extensive and constantly expanding. Several West End colleagues, Dr Borland for one, advised their patients to go to her when they themselves retired. Her reputation as a physician with an outstanding gift for diagnosis, and also as a charming person, was becoming widely known, for by now she had mastered the delicate art of combining the doctor–patient relationship with cordial personal friendships. Among her patients were quite a number of public figures, and she had many devotees in the circles that she nicknamed 'Debrett'.

One of the patients who had come to rely implicitly on her expertise was an elderly Scotswoman, Lady Jane Lindsay, daughter of the 25th Earl of Crawford and Balcarres, and Margery was on happily friendly terms with the vivacious Lady Jane – the portrait of her by de Laszlo shows a lively old lady with silvery hair and a countenance full of grace.

For some years before the war Lady Jane had lived in London, not far from Thurloe Street, and her house in Egerton Gardens had been a centre for a circle of friends who shared her interest in the arts. She was a spirited conversationalist, well-read and with a keen and inquiring mind, while at the same time she was a devout Christian, with an effusively affectionate nature which won friends for her everywhere.

When the war came her London house was requisitioned and she moved to the country, to stay for the duration with the widowed daughter-in-law of one of her sisters. This niece by marriage, Beatrice Majendie, lived in Essex, at Hedingham Castle near Halstead, and Lady Jane was already well acquainted with her home, a Queen Anne mansion which had been in the Majendie family for a century (formerly it belonged to the Earls of Oxford).

The house stands in surroundings of great beauty. Set high above an ornamental lake, it faces south and in fine weather it seems to bask in the sun; around it stand magnificent trees – cypresses, ilexes, maples, and a fantastic tulip tree which is said to be one of the largest in Britain, while nearby, across a Tudor bridge, towers 'the Keep', the remaining part of the Norman castle which gives Hedingham its name.

Before Lady Jane came to Hedingham in 1939 the atmosphere in the Majendie home had been cheerless, to say the least. Mrs Majendie was retiring in temperament, and because of ailing health she had long been leading the life of an invalid. Her husband had died some years earlier, and of her two sons one was in the Navy and the other in Africa. The only member of the younger generation living at home was her daughter Musette, then forty-two, who owing to her mother's incapacity had shouldered the responsibilities of running the Hedingham estate and acting as a leader in local affairs. But for much of the time she devoted herself unstintingly to caring for her mother, whom she adored.

Musette was an unusual and paradoxical person. In looks strongly built, with well defined features and a habitually firm expression, she had a voice which was singularly deep. She relished country activities – hunting, shooting, wooding – and was also energetically public-spirited. Since her youth she had been a leader in the Boy Scout movement (she had been awarded its highest honour, 'The Silver Wolf') while in the 1930s her work for the young unemployed had been recognised by the award of the CBE. But at the same time she was reserved, sensitive, very kind, and a nature lover. The sad family situation weighed heavily on her, taking its toll of her health, and leading her into a state of depression verging on breakdown, though she was able to find enjoyment in riding and also in driving – at one time she owned a Bugatti.

So it was indeed a blessing when Lady Jane, with her energy and sparkle and her loving temperament, arrived on the scene, especially as she was very fond of her great-niece. Predictably Musette became profoundly dependent upon 'Aunt Jeanie', and the two women, in spite of the discrepancy in their ages, were soon intimate friends. Especially after Musette's mother died, early in 1944, the two were constantly together. So much so that Lady Jane, by this time in her eighties, anticipated with dread the prospect that after her own death her beloved Musette would be left friendless and stranded.

This was how things stood when, in the autumn of 1945, Margery for the first time visited Hedingham. One weekend Lady Jane had been unwell, and she invited Margery to come and see her in the country and to stay overnight. So there were plenty of opportunities for Musette to become acquainted with her, and Lady Jane later wrote that this visit was 'a great turning point' in the lives of all three of them, for within the encounter there immediately emerged a remarkable affinity. During the ensuing months the friendship blossomed: both Lady Jane and Musette became Margery's devoted admirers, and Margery responded glowingly to their affection. On the anniversary of their fateful first meeting Lady Jane wrote to Margery:

> A year ago we came together for the first time. The thought of it moves me deeply. It was a vivid object lesson of God's watchful care for us.
>
> We all three had need of each other. It gave me – or rather has

since given me – an ever increasing thankfulness, having removed the dread I had felt of leaving her alone, objectless, and oh *so* lonely when I go! And now, witnessing the devoted tenderness of Musette for you and your great tender love for her, I cannot tell you the sweetness of my joy.

For I love you my Margery with all my heart quite apart from gratitude on behalf of what you have and always will do for us. But just because you *are* one of the sweetest, most lovable, finest creatures straight from Heaven.

Margery had evidently returned often to Essex during the early months of her friendship with Musette, for by the end of January 1946 she was referring to Hedingham as home. By then, too, she was calling Lady Jane 'Aunt Jeanie'. It seems clear that for Margery her loving friendship with Lady Jane and Musette was indeed a godsend, for it helped to fill the great gap in her life left by the death of Dr Campbell Morgan.

But one may well ask how Margery's new way of life affected her intimate association with Helena Banks, which had previously been so exclusive. Undeniably it caused difficulties, but Dr Banks, with her characteristic unselfishness, rose above the inevitable temptation to jealousy. A few years after Margery's first visit to Hedingham, Musette, in her generous way, lent to Dr Banks for her lifetime a charming cottage called the Garden House at the edge of the estate, so that she could use it as a 'holiday home' either for herself when she needed a rest or for relatives or patients. It was a great joy to her to be able to keep in touch with Margery at Hedingham without interfering with the life she shared with Musette. Dr Banks was more at home in the simple, peaceful surroundings of the cottage than in the busy and more formal atmosphere of the Castle.

Meanwhile, after the death of Beatrice Majendie the heavy death duties meant that at first it seemed doubtful whether Musette could afford to stay on at Hedingham. But largely thanks to an idea of Lady Jane's a viable way of running the vast house was found. Why not convert it into a place where elderly friends and relations could live their last years in a congenial atmosphere, or recuperate after illness, sharing Musette's home with her, and contributing to the running expenses?

Lady Jane herself had decided that she did not wish to return to London. She said that she wanted to spend her last days at Hedingham, and thus she set an example that many were to follow during the coming years. Musette, helped by Margery, tackled the problems of reorganising the interior of the house, with the addition of bathrooms so as to provide self-contained flats, and not long after Lady Jane died, in January 1948, the new regime was under way.

The aim was to create a friendly 'family' atmosphere with the highest standard of amenities. Obviously there would be a certain amount of coming and going, for some people would want to stay for a limited time, to convalesce or rest, while others, like Lady Jane, might want to end their lives at Hedingham.

At the start all the residents were women; a few men and married couples came later. Several of the earliest comers were relatives of Musette's; one of them was Lady Maud Erskine, a talented amateur artist who endeared herself to everyone – she was especially kind to new arrivals. Margery once said that she was the nicest person ever to come and live at Hedingham. But not all the residents were gregarious. For instance there was Miss Eva Tenison, an erudite historian, who most of the time shut herself into her book-lined room writing.

Many of Margery's patients settled down happily, and benefited much from their stay. For instance old Mrs Violet Boyle, who suffered from heart trouble. Before Margery took her on she had been told she had only a year to live, but after her move to Hedingham, in 1952, she lived contentedly on, under Margery's constant care, for twenty-two years; she died at the age of ninety-four. Another of the residents who spent her last years at Hedingham, loved by all, and who finally died there, was Lady Dorothy Meynell, a cousin of Musette's.

During Margery's second year as President of the Faculty she was admonished by Sir John Weir. Kensington was no place for an eminent physician to practise, he told her; she must certainly come to the Harley Street area. So for a time, after this, she did have a Wimpole Street address. But she never felt settled there, and she was soon back in Thurloe Street, happy to be once more on her home ground. There she had first found her feet as a general practitioner and there she meant to continue. There, for over twenty years, she had been receiving her patients and prescribing for them, gradually accumulating the experience that was making her into the most outstanding homoeopathic GP of her generation – a GP who could often tell at a glance which remedy was the right one for each particular man, woman or child.

The Thurloe Street house suited her to perfection. And, especially in her consulting room, she had created an atmosphere that reflected her personality. It was a pleasant ground-floor room, with windows facing south at the rear of the house. The only drawback was that the outlook was almost directly on to South Kensington underground station, with the recurrent rumble of passing trains. But this did not seem to intrude on the elegant interior, where long curtains in shades of pink harmonised with the brocade of the big couch with its immaculate linen spread, while a leather-covered screen embossed in mellow glowing colours hid the hand-basin and rows of medicines, neatly arranged in alphabetical order. Margery's desk was a ship's chest that had belonged to the Blackie family, and there was a big armchair for the patient, but the other furniture showed her taste for delicacy of style; a small Sheraton-type cabinet was fitted up for medicines, and a pair of Hepplewhite chairs were upholstered in Regency pin-striped material. The focal point in the room was always a shallow bowl filled with little flowers from Hedingham – 'a miniature garden' – so charmingly arranged by Dr Banks that patients could not fail to express delight. Margery had found that this helped them to relax. Another detail which added to the ambience of calm was the open fire, with logs from Hedingham.

Margery's patients, when asked for their memories of Thurloe Street, always speak of the flowers, in the waiting room as well as on Margery's desk. One lady has set down a delightfully spontaneous account of her visits to 'Dr Margery's private clinic', and has also added her grateful memories of Margery herself. 'She was a living example of how life should be lived, how folk should be treated and how money should be handled.' As a child, this lady remembered, she had been taken regularly by her mother to the London Homoeopathic Hospital, but before long she was being brought to Thurloe Street, where in those early days the fee was 'five shillings per examination'.

> You were shown into a warm, inviting waiting room, with a lovely log fire and a drift of delicate perfume from a dish in the centre of the table, which held a fantastic array of country flowers. It was a very homely place, where you were made to feel important just being 'You'.
>
> After waiting for your turn, Dr Blackie would open the door and say 'Come along now', in her dear old-fashioned way. She was a sweet-faced lady, always very smart, with a hint of the Victorian days. She had high necks to her blouses or jumpers, and a simple hair style taken back into a bun, but with soft waves at the front, and a very charming smile.
>
> Her consulting room will forever remain in my mind. It was beautifully furnished with antique furniture; a lovely open fireplace with brasses of a bygone age, a screen across the wash-basin area . . . and long curtains at the window trying to shut out the railway, which ran almost beneath the window. Her words after examination will ever ring in my ears: 'Oh! poor girl, never mind, we will soon put things right'.

An important part of Margery's practice was visiting her patients in their homes when necessary. She and Dr Banks shared a car, and 'Banks' who was a good and careful driver often took the wheel, so that Margery could rest, and perhaps doze, en route. This same patient remembers that when she was laid up and 'Dr Margery' came to her home, she always brought a small bunch of her 'home-grown flowers'.

Another woman patient, an academic, recalls that coming to consult Dr Blackie was like visiting a welcoming home. 'My first visit was in early March. I was shown into the dining room; on the oak table in the middle of the room stood a round bowl filled with heathers, mosses and small spring flowers. Waiting in that room was an aesthetic pleasure.' Then Margery herself came in and conducted her into the adjoining room, 'her own room, warmed by a bright fire'.

Dr Blackie was a small, spare woman who struck me as having immense but controlled energy. A warm handshake followed by a few words to put me at my ease and then, sitting very upright at her desk, paper and pen at the ready, she listened with interest, but not without the occasional serious or humorous interjection, to all I had to say. Everything was written down. Her main aim – in my case – was reassurance; explanations were not given till later, and the Latin name of the remedy was not translated into English.

There was, during the consultation, no sense of hurry, and if, in the course of it, a patient happened to ring up asking for advice, then advice was freely given. When this, my first interview, came to an end, Dr Blackie administered a soothing powder and said goodbye with a firm handshake. My first impression, of having been in contact with a most capable physician, was confirmed during subsequent visits, when I was made to feel equally welcome.

For Margery, despite her added responsibilities as President of the Faculty, the first priority was always her clinical work, both in the out-patient department at the hospital and at Thurloe Street. And meantime, during her years as President she showed her flair for inspiring leadership by championing the cause of the general practitioner. She became so firmly convinced that the future of homoeopathy in Britain depended upon the training of GPs, in other words the winning over of doctors who were already qualified in medical-school medicine, that among her colleagues the GP became known as 'Dr Blackie's hobby-horse'. 'The life of the general practitioner is hard but after twenty-five years of it I can't think of a better,' she insisted. 'The place where homoeopathy is most needed and can be most effective is in general practice. If only we could convert an army of young men and set them up in general practice there would no longer be any question of the survival of homoeopathy – it would spread in an incredible way.'

She was well aware of a growing demand for homoeopathic treatment. When she gave a lecture in Bournemouth to an audience of about two hundred, she was told afterwards that there was room for two or three homoeopaths in the area. This was very gratifying, of course, but it gave rise to a grave danger. For it was obvious that if the need for qualified homoeopaths in general practice was not met, there was bound to be a great increase in the number of lay practitioners, unqualified self-styled 'homoeopathic specialists', some of whom (in the words of a leading Scottish homoeopath, Dr Thomas Douglas Ross) were 'very ignorant and dangerous quacks'.

In Margery's third presidential address, in 1951, she underlined the need for homoeopathic GPs by recalling a remarkable case which she herself – as a visiting GP – had treated. It had been the sort of case, she said, that makes even a homoeopathic family more convinced and enthusiastic than ever. A girl of nineteen had come to London from Wales for a dance. The friends she was staying with disapproved of homoeopathy, but when next morning her temperature was soaring they telephoned, reluctantly, to Margery.

> I found her looking and feeling very ill, congested, and with a thickly coated tongue, severe headache, bad cough and feeling very sick. She improved slightly after *Byronia* [white bryony] and her temperature was lower in the evening. Next morning she was

coming out in a rash and by evening she had the thickest measles rash I have ever seen. I gave her *Sulphur* and she quickly improved and an early patch of congestion [in her lung] disappeared. Her father came by car at the end of a week and drove her back to Wales. And she went off to Yorkshire for another dance three days later.

Everyone was much impressed, Margery added, because four of the girl's friends had caught measles on the same day from the same contact, and they had been extremely ill – two had developed pneumonia. All four were still in bed when she went off to Yorkshire.

In this same presidential address she related some brief case histories to show that although a long first consultation is the norm in homoeopathic practice, an experienced GP can often judge what is needed on the spur of the moment. 'Prescribing homoeopathically is rather like bird watching,' she said. 'To begin with you study the flight, the size, the colour, the markings and all the rest, and then have to go to some book. But when you've been at it some time, one glance, with scarcely a thought, and you can name the bird. That doesn't come, though, without much experience and study.'

In a certain village where she was 'fairly well known,' she said, she often prescribed after only a few minutes' conversation in the street.★ She found that when she said 'Good morning, Mrs Smith, how are you?' this was not taken as a salutation but as an opportunity to describe a malady in the hope of being given a box of pills. There was no time to go into the case thoroughly, but Margery's spontaneous prescribing often produced astonishing results – in the case of Mrs H, for instance. She and her husband had been given notice to quit, after being in the same cottage for thirty-three years. She developed acute depression and a congestive early morning headache. *Natrum muriaticum* was given and within a week she was quite a different person – headache and depression gone.

★ She was obviously referring to Castle Hedingham.

Then there was Mrs K, who was thinking of changing her job. She loved cooking but thought that the heat and the standing were giving her rheumatism. She had pains in her wrist one day, in her knees the next, and all worse in bed at night. A very few days after being given *Pulsatilla* she had no more pains and there was no more talk of changing her job. Another time Margery asked Mrs R how her daughter was getting on; she knew the girl well. All right, her mother said, except that she was getting one stye after another. Again Margery prescribed *Pulsatilla*, and a fortnight later she was not surprised to hear that there had been no more styes. One day Mrs M asked Margery if she would see her husband. He had had an operation and could not pick up and was very worried about himself. He said he felt giddy and very scared several times a day, with sweating and nausea. Margery gave him *Arsenicum album* in a high potency, followed by low-potency *Arnica*, and when she saw him in the street ten days later he looked a different man. He was delighted with the improvement he had made in a week. Mrs C reported that she had sprained her ankle, and it was so painful that she would not be able to carry on. After some *Arnica* she was able to go to work next day. Old Mrs H, hobbling along when she met Margery, poured out the story of her bad varicose veins and cramps she had every night. In the past she had been helped by *Cuprum arsenicosum* (arsenite of copper) and she asked for some more as it had been marvellous.

Margery's final speech as President of the Faculty was her Valedictory Address. It was a vehement speech, strong, almost aggressive – a rousing challenge. 'What is our object as a faculty?' she demanded. 'What do we set out to do? We have monthly meetings [but] . . . out of 237 members the average attendance is twenty-five. I wonder why this ten per cent attend? Is it to pool experiences and learn from them or to give or get encouragement . . . or are these meetings just something to be endured from a sense of duty?' Then she spoke of the meetings she had attended when she was first at the hospital.

> We residents looked forward to them and they provided us with food for thought and discussion for the following week or two. We enjoyed the inevitable wordy battles between the high and low potency prescribers. We learned to know the hobby-horses and their riders . . . The fun was fast and sometimes furious, but . . . we residents came away encouraged and filled with fresh enthusiasm. Not only at the meeting, but around the tea table before and the dinner table after, homoeopathy was the only topic.

Then she turned to the contemporary situation. 'Do we have the same effect today on the beginner?' she asked. 'Is it because the results they have seen or heard about have failed to impress them, or have we failed to give them a real picture of what homoeopathy can do?'

> Last year I said that if homoeopathy was to spread and not merely to survive it was essential that we should have more and more homoeopathic general practitioners and I now repeat it . . . The duty of the Faculty is to provide the doctors. I feel we have sadly failed in the last three years, in spite of enquiries at lectures, week-end courses and at Faculty meetings. Books and lectures are essential, but something else is needed; the encouragement and enthusiasm which only personal contact can provide.

She spoke from the heart, and it is clear that the 'sad failure' of those three years was the impetus that spurred her to the personal efforts which were soon to transform the outlook for British homoeopathy. 'If I felt that I had impressed on my fellow members of the Faculty their responsibility in this matter,' she concluded, 'I'd feel that my presidency had not been in vain. My hobby-horse must certainly be called the General Practitioner and I hope he'll prove a winner in the not too distant future.'

Classical Homoeopathy

Her Majesty Queen Elizabeth II, youthful and radiant, made an official visit to the Royal London Homoeopathic Hospital during her third year on the throne. In 1955 the bicentenary of the birth of Samuel Hahnemann was being celebrated, and the Queen's visit, which took place on 10 November, emphasised her personal adherence to the Hahnemann tradition – to classical homoeopathy – the therapy which had helped so many of her relatives, especially her father. And indeed she herself, ever since childhood, had been accustomed to taking homoeopathic remedies.

While she toured the hospital, members of the staff were presented to her, and in the stately boardroom, with its portraits of the great ones of homoeopathy – Hahnemann, Quin, Clarke – one of the doctors who was brought forward was Dr Margery Blackie, by now a member of the hospital's management committee, as well as physician in charge of out-patients. This was Margery's first meeting with the monarch who fourteen years later was to become her patient.

A highlight of the day was when the royal visitor accepted, with obvious delight, the gift of a very remarkable bouquet. It was composed of forty-two kinds of flowers, berries, and plants, all of which are used to provide homoeopathic remedies. They included salvia, rosemary, iris, marigold, valerian, mimosa, laurustinus, snowberry, stinging nettle, clematis, spindleberry, plantain, Christmas rose. And needless to say, the beautiful mass of little flowers and plants, multicoloured and fragrant, had been arranged with exquisite skill by Helena Banks.

The Hahnemann bicentenary was also celebrated in the United States, where a group of devotees, centring round the American Institute of Homoeopathy, had organised a conference in Washington DC. Britain was represented by Sir John Weir (who after the death of King George VI had been appointed Physician to the new Queen). It was an impressive occasion, but there was no disguising the sad state of affairs in America as a whole. Homoeopathy had been taken over by its enemies and thereby emasculated. Although the American Institute of Homoeopathy had been founded in 1844, the very same year in which Quin had formed the British Homoeopathic Society, twentieth-century America had no equivalent to Britain's Faculty, teaching was in eclipse, and research, too, had dwindled almost to a standstill. In the early days, until the First World War, there had been many homoeopathic colleges, but these had gradually closed down owing to the manoeuvres of the medical establishment. Furthermore by Margery's time there were no leaders of the stature of the great Dr Kent to uphold the standards of classical homoeopathy in the research field.

Thus it had fallen to Britain to take the lead both in teaching and in research, the latter consisting chiefly of provings, the tests upon which classical homoeopathy had always depended, ever since Hahnemann first 'proved' his reactions to quinine. And here it may be mentioned that the unique value of this method of research, based on recordings of the effects which regulated doses of medicinal substances have had upon healthy individuals, lies in the fact that the volunteers, being articulate, can describe the nature of their reactions, sometimes slight, but more often acutely painful and distressing. Who are the men and women who willingly accept such sufferings in the interest of bringing healing to others? Over the years innumerable anonymous enthusiasts, many of them students at the Missionary School of Medicine, have come forward to offer themselves as guinea pigs. What a testimony of devotion!

Within the Faculty Margery served on the committee for research and drug proving, as well as on the committee for education; she was also, by the 1950s, not only a fellow and a council member, but for a year she was editor of the *British Homoeopathic Journal*. This latter position was potentially one of considerable influence, for the journal was the official mouthpiece of the Faculty. But literary work was not in Margery's line. Three issues appeared during her time but she wrote only one editorial (October 1955) and it was a perfunctory review of the current situation in medicine which had evidently been composed in a hurry. We may guess that she was missing the assistance of Dr Banks who at this time became gravely ill – stricken by poliomyelitis. Hitherto she had usually turned to her for help in the matter of lectures and speeches. Dr Banks's illness was also, obviously, a very serious blow to the Thurloe Street practice. She recovered to a certain extent, but was never able to resume her full-time partnership. She still helped Margery in many ways, such as dealing with telephone calls, but it was soon clear that the practice would have to enlist the help of other homoeopaths.

At about the time of Margery's resignation as editor of the *British Homoeopathic Journal*, it began to promote views which to her, and to other proponents of classical homoeopathy, were nothing less than heretical, for they questioned the pure and simple principles of Hahnemann. Doubt was thrown, for instance, upon one of his fundamental axioms, the validity of provings, on grounds that as there was no acceptable definition of 'a healthy individual' the whole proving experiment was based on unreliable premises.

But this irreverent attitude towards Hahnemann was not the only reason why Margery and others felt disturbed by the journal's 'new look'. Prominence was also being given to the metaphysical teachings of Rudolf Steiner, whose 'spiritual science' – anthroposophy – was in Margery's view anti-Christian.* She felt it was profoundly dangerous by reason of its occultism, and Musette agreed with her categorically on this point.

Margery had reason to know something about anthroposophy at first hand because of its strong influence upon two of her cousins, younger sisters of Ivy Compton-Burnett. Vera and Juliet Compton-Burnett had been so deeply involved that in 1949 they had taken on the running of the Rudolf Steiner school at King's Langley in Hertfordshire. But there was an earlier, much earlier, link, a skeleton in the family cupboard. At the time when Margery was starting as a medical student, Ivy Compton-Burnett's two youngest sisters, Primrose and Katharine ('Topsy'), almost exactly her contemporaries, whose mental balance had been impaired under the influence of 'mystical' teachings akin to anthroposophy, committed suicide by overdosing themselves with veronal. The shock and horror of this happening and the ensuing publicity may well have imbued Margery with a revulsion against all kinds of 'mystical' cults.

But she was not entirely consistent as regards anthroposophical medicine. One of Steiner's main endeavours in the medical field had been research into the treatment of cancer by means of a preparation of mistletoe known as *Iscador*. Injections of this liquid preparation were held, by his followers, to possess extra-ordinary powers – a belief that Margery could hardly be expected to share. Yet she did not refrain from prescribing *Iscador* occasionally, if she felt it might benefit a

* A definition of anthroposophy is given in the *Oxford Dictionary of the Christian Church* (1958, p. 61). It is described as 'a religious system evolved by R. Steiner from neo-Indian theosophy, but placing man instead of God in its centre. It aims at leading man by a certain discipline of "concentration" and "meditation" towards an "intuition" in which the lower ego received the vision of the higher self. Anthroposophy teaches a highly elaborated and fantastic doctrine of the origin of the world, the various epochs of mankind, the "sun being" ("*Sonnenwesen*") Christ, reincarnation, and "Karma". It has found adherents in Germany as well as in Britain and America, especially among those in search of religious experiences outside the normal channels of Church life.'

patient. There had been quite convincing trials, particularly in Germany, which proved that it had a distinct, though mild, anti-tumour effect, and this was probably why she decided to use it.

Margery often enlivened her lectures with striking metaphors, and on one occasion in the 1950s she drew upon her lifelong interest in birds. She spoke of 'the rapidly enlarging aviary' of modern medicine, which was having a 'mesmerising effect', and she likened 'the glamour of the antibiotics, anti-histaminics [*sic*] and the rest' to foreign birds about which little was so far known. 'One hears of their marvellous performances but often in a few months you hear more of their vicious tendencies and we await with interest every new discovery about them. While doing this, we seem to have become almost a little ashamed of our quiet, harmless, homely little sparrow, homoeopathy, about which we know so much and which has been tried and proved over the last 160 years and not found wanting.'

The decade after the Second World War was certainly a time of brave new developments in medicine. Reliance was being placed more and more upon the newly discovered 'wonder drugs', despite their alarming side-effects – or more explicitly their poisonous effects. This was, of course, many years before thalidomide. The sulfa drugs and penicillin were saving many lives, but the majority of patients, after being given medication with certain other drugs, complained that the treatment made them feel worse than the disease. Furthermore it was being said that modern medicine was becoming more and more a system of suppression – of sweeping the dust under the mat – and that most of the new remedies do not cure, they merely relieve. This situation was indeed becoming such a commonplace to the medical profession that a new word, 'iatrogenic', had to be coined to describe the ills caused by the use of the 'wonder drugs'. In contrast to this, as one of Margery's colleagues, Dr Kathleen Priestman, has pointed out, all homoeopathic physicians are familiar with the phrase 'I feel so much better in myself' spoken by a smiling patient after the right homoeopathic remedy has taken effect. It was hardly surprising that among homoeopaths the general attitude to the new drugs was one of suspicion.

Nevertheless, as Margery herself realised, there were certain occasions, for example critical moments in illnesses such as meningitis where life was at risk, when it was imperative to resort to the antibiotics. At such moments it might be impossible to find the right 'homoeopathic arrow' with the necessary degree of certainty, and then the use of an 'orthodox blunderbuss' such as penicillin was entirely justified. The new 'lethal weapons' could not be ignored. And among the classical homoeopaths, led of course by Margery, the idea began to grow that homoeopathic medicines and antibiotics could and should, in some instances, work together.

Meanwhile in one respect medical-school medicine itself was veering towards the homoeopathic principle of like curing like. The prophylactic 'shot' (in which a very small quantity of a toxic substance akin to the disease is injected) was by now accepted by the general public as a matter of course, not only in the case of vaccination, and immunisation against diphtheria, measles, and other common diseases, but particularly for travellers going abroad to countries where they might be exposed to cholera, yellow fever, etc. Thus the advance of medical science was providing the very strongest confirmation of the natural law upon which homoeopathy is based. Unwittingly the upholders of non-homoeopathic medicine were themselves adopting in practice the principle which in theory they rejected with ridicule.

In 1957, when Margery was approaching the age of sixty, she became a consultant physician at the Royal London Homoeopathic Hospital. And when, two years later, she delivered the annual Richard Hughes Memorial Lecture, the President of the Faculty, Dr William Thomson Walker, said that there was no need to introduce the lecturer: 'Dr Margery Blackie is the best known and possibly the best loved of all the present consultants at the hospital.' Furthermore, he said, the audience was anxious to hear her, 'for she has given racy lectures in the past'. This was quite true, and it is interesting to realise that her 'raciness' can be attributed basically to her firm belief that empirical evidence was infinitely more important than 'scientific proof'. For she always included many case histories in her lectures and she recounted them in an anecdotal fashion that made for enjoyable listening.

When she gave her Richard Hughes lecture some of her audience may well have thought it ironic that she should have been invited to celebrate the memory of a renowned homoeopath who was famous for his advocacy of the 'scientific approach', since in her earliest days as a doctor she had been a disciple of the great Dr Clarke, and from him she had learnt to regard the search for a 'scientific meeting ground' with the critics as almost a betrayal of pure homoeopathy, a denial that clinical evidence – the evidence that 'it works' – is the only needful vindication.

In her lecture Margery admitted that Hughes claimed to be a faithful follower of Hahnemann. Having found the truth and advantages of the homoeopathic principle, she said, his chief desire was that everyone should benefit from it in its purest form (he even went so far as to call non–classical homoeopaths 'mongrels'). Yet he believed that there must be some modification of the way in which homoeopathy was presented, a way more in tune with 'the advances of modern investigation', which would avoid exciting 'repugnance or contempt' in the disciples of the scientific medicine of the day. What he meant by this was that an answer to the question 'How does homoeopathy work?' must be given in the language of science, rather than in the form of evidence which scornful critics could dismiss as 'mere anecdotes'.

Hughes was very keen to interest 'the orthodox medicals', as he called them, in the Hahnemann method. He sought 'to harmonise classical homoeopathy with general medicine'. In his own words, 'What medicine might become in ten years, if only the profession at large would test homoeopathy as it deserves, is a dream almost too bright to dwell on.' Margery's comment on this outburst was curt: 'We still have those among us today who hope and dream and work for this harmony. But I think history has proved them wrong . . . Prejudice is as deeply rooted in the medical profession today as it was then . . . If Hughes failed with all his zeal and enthusiasm, in a day when the newness of the method made a great impact . . . how can we in this day of wonder drugs hope to succeed? . . . I am sure the pure Hahnemannian prescribers will always remain few in number; the extra learning and work necessary will only appeal to the doctor whose chief interest is in the well being of the patient himself, rather than in the disease.'

Yet in this matter of the empirical versus the scientific Margery herself was not entirely consistent. In spite of her straight speaking in the Richard Hughes lecture her thinking was beginning to change. In spite of the influence of Dr Clarke and of her own convictions she was coming to realise that the evidence of clinical reports alone would never win over the unbelieving opposition. And already in certain ways she was actually co-operating with 'the scientists'. For many years she had gladly supported the work of Dr William Boyd of Glasgow, Britain's leading researcher into the 'secrets' of homoeopathy, by helping to organise fund-raising events in aid of the Boyd Medical Research Trust. The first of these had been the Myra Hess recital in 1947. And then in 1954 another occasion, on a more ambitious scale, took place at Hedingham: a 'Grand Ball', with a champagne supper at midnight and dancing in the Norman keep till 3 a.m. But the Hedingham ball was not exclusively in aid of Dr Boyd's work. It was also in aid of the Homoeopathic Research and Educational Trust, which had been established in London in 1948, as a registered charity, to raise and administer funds for the work of the Faculty.

Margery's dedication to her practice as a doctor was by no means the full extent of her work for the homoeopathic cause. She was an inspiring organiser. She was not a 'business woman', but with her dynamic energy, her burning enthusiasm, and also with her 'style' – her friends often use this word to describe her – she achieved successes where many a business woman would have failed.

Town and Country

As she entered her sixties Margery did not look anything like her age. She might well have been ten years younger. Not a wrinkle, a complexion still fresh, laughing eyes, only a touch of silver in her soft wavy hair. Her erect posture too was that of a young woman. A friend had said 'the straight back was characteristic; one would have thought she had been a rider all her life'.

Furthermore her style of dressing was timeless. By now she had developed a philosophy of dress. She believed that it was part of her job to look smart and cheerful. And she was fortunate in finding a couturier who perfectly understood her, namely Mr Peter Crown of Lachasse. He helped her to develop her own special style, an attractive style which made a lasting impression on colleagues and patients alike. She knew exactly what suited her and kept to it. Mr Crown recalls that when he showed her his new models she made decisions with the utmost speed, and she did not change her mind afterwards. She liked neat, softly tailored suits; her daytime clothes had to be functional and a little formal but at the same time feminine. For the evening however she chose 'classical romantic' gowns.

Margery had very definite preferences as regards colour. 'Autumn colours' were some of her favourites – topaz, mustard, banana, aubergine. She also loved a vivid cyclamen pink and occasionally chose a bright green though never blue. But her 'primary colour' was red – so much so that one of her patients used to refer to her in fun as 'the Red Queen'. Another patient, whom she visited often at home in the early days at

Thurloe Street, has told that in winter Margery always wore a big cape, and 'at all seasons very sensible flat shoes'. But in contrast to the shoes she sometimes appeared in exotic hats, 'all feathers and ribbons'. Apparently it was only in later years that she came to prefer a classic style in millinery.

The date of Margery's birth was something she preferred not to mention, but in her professional life it could not be kept secret, for at sixty-five she was officially due for retirement. It was unthinkable however that 'Blackie' should abandon her life's work when she was still at the height of her powers. At a meeting of the management committee of the Royal London Homoeopathic Hospital in April 1962 it was 'strongly recommended' that she should continue on the staff, and this she did for several years. And although in the spring of 1965 her out-patient work came to an end, in the following year, when she was sixty-eight, she was given the rank of honorary consultant.

A period of intense activity began for Margery after she had passed the normal retirement age. Her work at the hospital, her care for her patients, her teaching work, her leadership in conferences, all these continued as usual, but in addition, some of her most notable achievements were in the field of fund-raising. The Homoeopathic Research and Educational Trust, upon which the Faculty depended for training and for research, is nowadays supported largely by grants from foundations, companies, and other corporate bodies, but in the past the money had to be raised almost entirely by the efforts of individuals. So there was ample scope for Margery to serve the cause by means of her flair for planning and organising. Her enthusiasm was irrepressible and infectious, and although her little handwritten notes inviting support, dashed off in an unceasing flow, were always charmingly worded, they were in fact commands.

In all her organising she worked very closely with Musette. They saw eye to eye, and decided everything personally, as they both abhorred committees (there had been a committee for Margery's earliest fund-raising event, the Myra Hess recital at Chelsea Town Hall, after which they both agreed 'never again').

Several of their joint enterprises in aid of the Trust were staged at Hedingham, where Musette's position as an Essex landowner meant that she was able to rope in impressive support from county notables. One of these events was a dress show in the spring of 1964, a project that sprang from Margery's cordial relationship with Lachasse. Musette too, through Margery's introduction, had become a Lachasse client, and Mr Crown himself, who always advised Margery, also looked after 'Miss Majendie', whom he admired for her amiable manner and her sense of humour. It may seem surprising that Musette, so essentially a countrywoman, should be dressed by one of the most exclusive fashion houses in London. For she was never happier than in shabby gardening clothes, with a shapeless hat crammed down on her head, or – best of all – in khaki scouting uniform.* But she realised that for Margery's sake she must sometimes dress up, and when she accompanied her on formal occasions she looked stately and dignified, though she always chose sombre colours – gray, brown, or black – for she liked to remain in the background. One of her sayings was 'Margery is the peacock'.

At the Hedingham dress show, Lachasse's spring and summer collection was shown, consisting of eighty-two suits, dresses and evening gowns. There were two showings, one in the afternoon and one in the evening. The Duchess of Gloucester, ever faithful in her support of homoeopathic causes, came by helicopter to open the afternoon show and was greeted by the Lord Lieutenant of Essex. Then to Musette's delight she inspected a boy-scout guard of honour. In the evening, after the Princess had left, the second showing was opened by one of the most beautiful and elegant of

* The dress show was not only in aid of the Homoeopathic Research and Educational Trust but for 'the furtherance of Scouting in Essex'.

Margery's patients, Lady Namier, the Russian widow of the historian Sir Lewis Namier.

This highly successful occasion was not the only fund-raising event at Hedingham that year. In June there was a Grand Ball in the Keep, on the same lines as the one that had been held ten years earlier. And subsequently, at a meeting of the Faculty, Margery triumphantly presented a cheque for the sum of five thousand pounds.

Hedingham was, by this time, as much Margery's home as Thurloe Street, for she was there every weekend, playing a leading part in the 'house party', which was now well established on the lines that 'Aunt Jeanie' had envisaged. Within the vast house, eight suites had been created for the residents – many of them widows and widowers – who could feel at home since they often brought with them their own pieces of furniture, rugs, pictures and books. But several of the spacious rooms on the ground floor were available to all, so that they could join in the pattern of life that centred round their two hostesses.

Musette and Margery took great pains to assess whether those who wanted to come to Hedingham would fit in, and usually all was well. One of Musette's relatives who thrived especially at Hedingham, and was dearly loved and respected by all, was Miss Alice Corry, a cousin of Lord Halifax. But not everyone took to the life. Mrs Norway, widow of the author Nevil Shute, did not stay long, nor did two of the married couples who came for trial periods.

Neither did everyone who seemed likely to be an ideal addition to the community respond as Margery hoped. In 1971 her patient Lady Namier, who since the death of her second husband had been living alone in her London flat, decided to withdraw to a home, and was making plans to go to a house in Surrey belonging to the Friends of the Elderly. When Margery learnt this she was shocked and disturbed, and she resolved to press her to change her mind. But Lady

Namier was a very decisive person, as is clear from some letters she wrote to a friend at the time. She told her that 'dear Blackie', who was due to give her a regular check-up, had heard of her intentions, and wanted to persuade her to transfer herself to Hedingham Castle instead of Coulsdon. 'I shall have to muster the strength to be firm without giving offence,' she wrote, 'not too easy.' A few days later she wrote again:

> My meeting with Blackie started badly. She sat despondent, repeating under her breath 'I can't bear it', i.e. my moving to Coulsdon. But when I was at last moved to ask what I would do at Hedingham if (which heaven forbid) I outlived both her and Musette, she pulled herself up with a jerk and energetically said 'What indeed!' The matter was closed, the ordeal over. What an intelligent woman! And so good in so many ways.

The matter was closed, but it left Margery despondent. Lady Namier's move to Coulsdon would mean losing touch with someone who was not only a patient but a dear friend.

From the domestic angle, the Hedingham establishment was run by a team consisting of a 'lady administrator', a butler, and relays of daily helpers – more than twenty of them. Village life centred round 'the Castle', and the people of the village all looked up to Musette, so the enlisting of help was no problem, and she in turn took a great pride in their standards. Meanwhile there was an outdoor staff of six. What a contrast to Margery's simple, cosy life with Helena Banks in London, where the only domestic was their faithful Irish cook-housekeeper 'Aggie' (Agnes Joyce), who was an intimate friend as well as a servant.

One may ask how such a grandiose scale of life was financed. Were all the residents millionaires? Not at all; but details of what they paid cannot be established because Musette and Margery used to decide, on an ad hoc basis, how much to charge in each case. There was no 'fixed charge'. And in order to avoid any odious comparisons, all the records were later destroyed. We do know, however, that at one time the

Hedingham estate included several farms, and these were gradually sold off. 'Hedingham worked well for a bit,' is the observation of one who was in a position to know, 'but it became hopelessly uneconomic business-wise.'

In addition to the residents, visitors often came to Hedingham for the day or for short periods, to rest or convalesce; Edith Sitwell was one of these, also Myra Hess and Dr Martyn Lloyd-Jones and his wife. For all of them, life was dominated by Musette, the benevolent autocrat. One of Margery's friends has jokingly said that Miss Majendie imposed martial law; 'you were told what to do.' This was true, and furthermore there were a number of conventions that had to be obeyed. When a certain lady, a newcomer, appeared wearing slacks Musette drew her aside and said firmly, 'We don't dress like that here.'

In the summer croquet was de rigueur, the hoops were set out on the lawn near the giant tulip tree. Margery herself became a very good player, but she did not like losing. Indoors, summer and winter, jigsaw puzzles were always on the go; for thirty years Margery subscribed to the British Jig-Saw Puzzle Library, and these puzzles were her favourite pastime, her greatest pleasure at weekends. Incidentally she found them therapeutic, for the concentration took her mind briefly away from her work. Musette was also a jigsaw enthusiast, and her method of finding a sequence was according to colours. Margery on the other hand worked according to shapes.

Everybody assembled for lunch and dinner in the dining room, where most of the residents had their own tables. Dinner was a formal occasion; the ladies always changed into long dresses and the men wore smoking jackets. Card games were an evening ritual except on Sundays, for Musette was a strict Sabbatarian. Margery much enjoyed bridge and was a good player, but as with croquet she did not like losing, and Musette tried to arrange that she should win.

Going off to bed was another ritual. The staff had departed

and 'goodnight drinks' had been left ready in thermos flasks. Margery always liked a very strong cup of tea, a habit from her hospital days. Then, for Musette and Margery, after the goodnights and before the devotional Bible reading with which they always ended the day, it was time for some light reading. Margery's favourite authors were Dickens, Jane Austen, Mrs Gaskell and Dorothy Sayers. Musette had other tastes; she preferred stories of courage and adventure. She was definitely a prude: 'disgusting' was her comment on anything to do with sex. It may be mentioned here that Margery, too, although professionally very understanding and helpful about marital problems and gynaecological matters, was likewise averse to discussing sexual behaviour. In the words of one of her patients: 'One always felt in her a source of joy and confidence and protection; I don't think there was a thing one couldn't discuss with Margery (except love affairs).'

No wonder that Hedingham brought about changes in Margery. One friend of hers maintains that the years she shared with Musette did much to 'educate' her, which is a way of saying that country life, and all that went with it, gave her a new poise, and brought out and enhanced her natural refinement. A patient who first consulted her in her Hedingham days once made a significant remark:'I thought that Dr Blackie came of an aristocratic family.' Another interesting point has been made by one of Margery's colleagues. He believes that her participation in the leisurely country-house life assisted her work in a subtle way: 'A lot of Margery's patients were country people, and the country rhythm at Hedingham helped her to understand them.' Yes, but it was a 'country rhythm' that had involved courageous self-sacrifice on Margery's part. Since she had been a town-dweller for so long, it had been something quite new for her to try to experiment in the riding, shooting, fishing and so on that were the norm at Hedingham, and she only made the effort to do so for Musette's sake.

At weekends Margery was supposed to be off duty, though in a sense she was never *not* 'on call'. If any of her patients wanted to see her urgently on a Saturday or Sunday her 'time off' was entirely forgotten. But normally, on Friday evenings, as Musette drove her out of London in one of the Hedingham cars (the 'fleet' consisted of at least three saloons, a station wagon and a Land Rover) her professional self was more or less left behind. Next Monday she would again be 'Blackie', the quick, decisive, aggressive chief known so well to her fellow doctors, and she would also be the 'Doctor Blackie' beloved by her patients, the gentle, compassionate physician, who always remembered the details of one's case, and prescribed with such utter confidence. But on Saturday and Sunday she could be herself, 'just Margery'. And for this reason the memories of those who knew her well at Hedingham are of outstanding interest, as evidence of what she was really like as a person.

Some of these memories show qualities, tastes and characteristics that might seem unexpected. People who met her casually tended to think of her as hard and brilliant. But behind this façade, so it appears, she was very vulnerable, and sensitive to the reactions of others. She thrived on affection, glowed in response to it, relished being appreciated.

Did she ever really 'unwind'? At Hedingham, yes, in certain ways. For one thing she was able to give herself up to bird-watching – hour after hour. She had always been fascinated by birds, even as a girl in a London suburb, and now, surrounded by forest trees and the thickets of the estate, she could develop her intimate understanding of them. With help from Musette, too, she learnt to recognise the different bird songs. She also enjoyed the ritual of the bird table outside the drawing-room window. No cats were allowed at Hedingham – for the sake of the birds. And in other ways, too, bird life was given precedence. There is a story that one day a shy visitor was trying to make conversation with Margery about gardening, and the subject of forsythia came up. 'What a problem the birds are, aren't they,' said the visitor, 'always pecking the buds off.' Quick as lightning came the reply: 'We grow the forsythias specially for them!'

Both Margery and Musette took a lively interest in the garden, but according to one of Margery's patients, whose husband was a real expert, they were erratic in their enthusiasm. He enjoyed giving them plants, but they generally put them in the wrong places. His wife, who was devoted to Margery, tells a tale that illustrates their misplaced zeal. Her husband once gave them a large crown imperial bulb, which excited them very much, and having planted it they poured over it a whole bottle of fertiliser. 'It grew and grew, like a young tree, and finally produced a head of so many huge flowers, not on stalks but bunched together, that it was a monster, a deformity, and they were astonished and rather discouraged.'

Margery loved flowers; gentians were her favourites while Musette preferred auriculas and lilies. But their main joy was in the water plants of a bog garden at the edge of the lake, which had been created by Musette's mother. They were often to be seen there together, paddling about in their wellingtons. A summerhouse nearby was one of the places where Margery often sat, and her pet robin would come flitting along to be fed with the worms she kept specially for him. But not all wild life appealed to her: she could not bear insects and was genuinely frightened of wasps, and creatures that she called 'creepy crawlies'.

Extremely direct in her likes and dislikes, she could on occasion be impatient and intolerant. On the subject of snowdrops she was once heard to say, 'I hate them! So often my fingers have been frozen when I had to pick the horrid little things!' And a friend remembers another time when Margery vented feelings of hate; this was in quite a different context. On Sunday mornings Margery always went to the Castle Hedingham parish church with Musette, who often read the lessons (she studied them beforehand and read them clearly and well).★ And on one occasion when they were returning after the service, as they passed the garden of some neighbours

★ Musette had inherited the patronage of the church and was its Lay Rector. Margery became joint patron with her.

they noticed that washing was hanging on the line. Shocked to the core Margery exclaimed, 'I *hate* them!'

Sunday lunch was always a special occasion. Wine was served for everyone; Margery's favourite was a very sweet Barsac. Musette and she sat at a big main table, with any visitors and friends; sometimes there were as many as sixteen at the 'high table'. The residents were all around at their smaller tables. Margery liked to be at the centre of conversation, and sometimes she would break in with a bombshell remark such as 'I hate ladybirds!' If the talk turned to politics she was frankly bored, unlike Musette who enjoyed expressing her extremely right-wing views. But if religion was discussed Margery had plenty to say. She did not hesitate to proclaim her distrust of Roman Catholicism. She declared that she was thankful for the discarding of 'papal trappings' at the Reformation. 'We had a wonderful Reformation to get rid of all those tendencies.'

But despite this prejudice a few of the Hedingham residents were Catholics. And sometimes Margery, after she had been 'true to herself' – in other words opinionated – in her remarks, realised that she had caused hurt feelings. Then, overcome with remorse, she would bow her head, and say softly to herself, 'I am condemned.' Truth was her ultimate value, but she was also intensely conscientious.

Country life for Margery meant Hedingham. She very seldom made the effort of getting away elsewhere, except sometimes in summer to Scotland. She was so utterly immersed in her work, in her teaching and planning, in her care for her patients, that she was virtually unable to cut herself off. Even when she did 'get away' she always took along a case of homoeopathic remedies, and she would pause en route if she happened to come into touch with someone who looked ailing.

The objective of the Scottish trips was a cottage in the Highlands, wonderfully situated at Pityoulish in the hills near Aviemore, in complete isolation and with magnificent views of the Spey valley. After Helena Banks recovered from polio, a patient, Henry Duckworth, had offered to lease this cottage to her, at a peppercorn rent, as a holiday retreat. When she first took on Milton Cottage it was a dreary brown croft, devoid of modern conveniences, but she had it painted white, put up yellow curtains, equipped it and made it charming.

Over the years Margery spent several holidays at Pityoulish. It was an ideal base for bird-watching, and for long walks when she eagerly sought out rare wild flowers. Musette, when she accompanied Margery to the cottage, enjoyed chopping wood for the open fire, and in the evenings, by lamplight, the two friends read the Bible together. This was the only sort of holiday Margery liked. Conventional 'social' holidays bored her stiff. There is a story that some friends once persuaded her to go abroad with them, to the South of France, for a break. She soon cabled to Helena Banks asking to be 'summoned back' to London.

PART THREE

First Lady

Royal Physician

A jubilee celebration, a splendid dinner at the Savoy Hotel in the presence of the Duke and Duchess of Gloucester, took place in honour of Sir John Weir in 1960, when he had completed fifty years of association with the Royal London Homoeopathic Hospital. He was then eighty-one, and it might well have been the moment to withdraw, in all the glory of royal congratulations and professional accolades. But he could not bring himself to give up, though he can hardly have been unaware of the general feeling among his colleagues, and among his patients too, that the time had come for him to resign his position as leading British homoeopath and physician to the royal family. The portrait of him by James Gunn which was unveiled that evening, and which in due course was hung in the hospital's boardroom, shows a genial but stubborn old man who was determined not to make way for anyone – least of all perhaps for Margery, who was his obvious successor.

There was no denying however that Sir John's tenacity and powers of endurance had brought about many triumphs for homoeopathy, not least in connection with his faithful service to the royal family. As long ago as 1918 he had attended King George V. Then in 1923 came his appointment as Physician-in-Ordinary to the Prince of Wales, and this did not end until the abdication. The Duke of York, before he succeeded his brother, was another of Weir's royal patients, and after his accession, as King George VI, he made Weir one of his official physicians. Throughout his reign Weir was his trusted adviser and friend.

Of course Sir John was only one of the doctors and surgeons who shared the grave responsibility of making decisions as regards the Monarch's health, but it was Weir who was often at the King's side, or chatting with him on the telephone. And the King's reliance upon him, as well as his belief in the efficacy of homoeopathic medicine, are indicated in a letter written from Sandringham on 3 February 1952, only three days before his death. The King said that he found it difficult to find adequate words in which to thank Sir John for 'all the wonderful help' he had given him 'during a friendship, a deep friendship, which began over thirty years ago.' His Majesty also said, in the same letter, 'I am a firm believer in your form of medicine, and it suits me.'

This moving tribute could have been echoed by several other members of the royal family. Queen Mary, for one, who had long known Weir through her husband, had appointed him as her own physician at the time of King Edward VIII's abdication, and for the next seventeen years, up until her death, she was an ardent enthusiast for homoeopathy. She not only relied on the remedies Weir prescribed, but also acquired a remarkable grasp of Hahnemann's teachings, and thoroughly enjoyed discussing them. It was through her that Princess Alice, the Duchess of Gloucester, soon after her marriage to Prince Henry, came to know about homoeopathy, for the young Duchess saw much of her mother-in-law.

Princess Alice first consulted Sir John in September 1936, and subsequently, over the years, she became the foremost royal supporter of homoeopathic occasions, gracing banquet after banquet and function after function with her presence. She also set an example by her confidence in the therapy, especially in homoeopathic 'first aid' – in *Arnica*, for instance, that outstandingly efficacious remedy for shock and bruises. In 1965, when she and her husband were preparing for a tour of Australia, they went to London by car for Winston Churchill's funeral, and on the return journey a terrible accident occurred. The Rolls swerved off the road and somersaulted three times. Miraculously Prince Henry escaped without serious injury, but Princess Alice suffered ghastly facial damage including a broken nose. An arm was also broken and a knee cracked. As she regained consciousness she kept saying '*Arnica, Arnica*'. But no one understood; they thought she was delirious. Then fortunately her maid came on the scene and she had some *Arnica* with her.

Later, in Bedford Hospital, the Princess had to have fifty-seven stitches in her face. But all were amazed at her rapid recovery, and before she left the hospital the Matron had given *Arnica* to other road-accident patients, who thereupon made 'magical' improvements. And the Duchess, in her *Memoirs*, has told that she was sufficiently well again in five weeks to accompany Prince Henry to Australia, where they arrived only one week later than had been originally planned.

At the time of the accident Weir was still the Princess's doctor, but she had already become acquainted with Margery, and eventually, even before Sir John finally retired, she wrote to her, on 1 October 1967, asking if she might be her patient. 'As you well know,' she wrote, 'I have for many years taken a great interest in homoeopathy and have great faith in the little pills which have always helped me so much.'

> Now that Sir John Weir has reached a great age I would not think it fair to call upon him for his advice as I know he would come at once and struggle up our long staircase and that would not be at all good for him at his age. I therefore write to ask if you would agree to be my homoeopathic adviser in his stead.
>
> Perhaps you would discuss this with Sir Ronald Bodley Scott* with whom I know you are well acquainted and I am sure he will know if there is anything more that we should do in regard to making this arrangement. I have just written to Sir John and told him that I am writing to you.

---

* Then Physician to HM the Queen.

Another member of the royal family who was to find Margery a worthy successor to Sir John was Queen Elizabeth the Queen Mother. In December 1967 she wrote to Margery from Clarence House, '. . . It was very nice that you were able to come yesterday with Sir John.' This shows that, despite Weir's jealous hold on his prerogatives, Margery was able to gain experience of attending upon royalty even before he retired – at long last – in 1968, at the age of eighty-nine.

The new year of 1969 was a time of ecstatic rejoicing for Margery's friends and patients, as well as for homoeopathic enthusiasts far and wide. For in the *London Gazette*, after the announcement of Sir John Weir's retirement from the Royal Medical Household, a second announcement was made by the Lord Chamberlain's office: 'The Queen has been graciously pleased to appoint Margery Grace Blackie, MD, MB, BS, MRCS, LRCP, FFHom, to be a Physician to Her Majesty.'

The torrent of congratulations was overwhelming. 'How happy dear Douglas Borland would have been,' wrote a long-time patient. 'So often we spoke about you . . . And now our dear loyal Queen has, thank God, chosen you. This will be a magnificent "uplift" for homoeopathy.'

She also received glowing letters from doctors who were not themselves homoeopaths – she often worked in co-operation with Harley Street specialists. The late Sir Ralph Marnham, the eminent surgeon, after offering his congratulations added, 'I also feel that I must take this opportunity of entirely dissociating myself from the ridiculous views attributed to the medical profession by the medical correspondents of the Daily Press. I suppose the poor so-and-so's must write something.'

Most of the reports of Margery's appointment were impartial, but in *The Times*, in the gossip column signed 'PHS', there was a malicious paragraph headed 'Woman Doctor for the Palace'.

> The new medical appointment to the Royal Household has come as a surprise to the medical profession. Not because Dr Margery

Blackie is a woman; indeed, there are not a few doctors – not all of them women or feminists – who have wondered for some time why there was no lady among the medical attendants of the royal family. Neither is it necessarily because she is so relatively unknown. Her name does not appear in *Who's Who*, and apart from her professional qualifications the only appointment shown against her name in the *Medical Directory* is that of consultant in general medicine to the Royal London Homoeopathic Hospital.

What has caused surprise is her age and the fact that she is a homoeopath – a section of the medical profession that one seldom hears of these days. Sir John Weir, of course, who has now retired at a ripe old age from his royal appointment, is the doyen of homoeopaths and there can be little doubt that his influence must have played a part.

But why someone so relatively old? To have qualified 45 years ago, as Dr Blackie did, means that she must be over 65, which is now recognized as the retiring age from medical appointments to the Royal Household.*

This wounding attack spurred several of Margery's patients to write in sympathy. Lady Namier wrote: 'I cannot refrain from adding my voice to the chorale of congratulations upon your appointment. I cannot refrain, because of the snide remarks in *The Times*. Always an envious hissing will do its best at a time like this. But it will die down somewhere over the bog where it started.'

As Lady Namier anticipated, the 'hissing' did die down, or rather it was silenced by the burst of acclamation that came to Margery, not only from people who knew her personally. 'We have never met,' wrote one correspondent from Pakistan, 'but your name is a world legend, your writings and articles have always been of the first order . . . Your appointment as a physician to HM the Queen is therefore not only a great honour to yourself, but also the greatest honour to the homoeopathic profession the world over.'

The manifest climax of Margery's career – a triumphant

* The writer seems to have been unaware that exceptions to the retirement-age rule are sometimes permitted.

event, a public proclamation of royal support for homoeo-pathy – took place in London, at the Guildhall, in the year following her appointment as Physician to the Queen. The occasion was an evening reception, a part of the 1970 British Homoeopathic Congress, of which Margery was President. There had been many such receptions before, but the 1970 reception was unique, because Her Majesty the Queen had graciously consented to be present.

For months beforehand Musette and Margery and a team of helpers were busy with the necessary formalities, for instance they had to approach the regimental headquarters of the Household Cavalry to ask for a band to play 'God Save the Queen', and in order to request the services of the State Trumpeters they had to get in touch with a gentleman known as the Silver-Stick-in-Waiting.

At last everything was ready, and at 8.45 on 22 October an assembly of nine hundred, the men in tails with decorations, the ladies in their evening best, awaited the arrival of Her Majesty. Sparkling with jewels, and wearing the sapphire-blue ribbon of the Garter, the Queen led a procession into the Guildhall, accompanied by the Lord Mayor of London in full regalia. Immediately after her came the Lady Mayoress with Margery, who was at her most elegant in a superbly simple gown of deep red double satin, with long white gloves.

When the time came for the presentations, Margery stood at the Queen's side, and introduced to her, one after another, Britain's leading homoeopaths. She also presented a number of others including general practitioners who were using homoeopathy more and more in their practices, as well as several benefactors of homoeopathy, and some visiting homoeopaths from Switzerland, Belgium, Finland, Greece, and the USA.

One of the letters she received after the reception enthused especially about Her Majesty: 'I expected the Queen to be gracious. I was not prepared for the extraordinary personal charm she possesses.' And another letter, more explosive in its appreciation, gave acclaim to Margery herself: 'What an evening! What an achievement! What a tribute to Dr Blackie!'

'She was an inspired teacher – you remembered the things she taught.' This simple but heartfelt tribute to Margery was made not long ago by a doctor who is now one of the best-known homoeopaths in Britain. Similar praise, in more flowery terms, had been offered to her by a young Indian woman. 'Indeed you are a great physician,' she wrote, 'but what is more important to me as a student is that you are a great teacher as well! The most fascinating, wonderful teacher I have ever had. Believe me, Dr Blackie, no student of yours can ever forget you. Most certainly I will not. You have opened new horizons for me.'

As a lecturer Margery had always been popular, because of her lively style and sense of humour. But during the mid-1960s her enthusiasm for the teaching of homoeopathy had begun to find new opportunities for expression; in 1964 she had been elected Dean of the Faculty of Homoeopathy. This meant that she was put in charge of the teaching policies which set the standards for Britain – and indeed, by means of the British lead, set an example to the whole world.

Ever since Quin's time teaching had been a major responsibility of the British Homoeopathic Society (and then of the Faculty) and for many years there had been annual lectures and also three-term courses for medical graduates. But in 1961 an additional project had been launched, in the form of short introductory courses for general practitioners. These 'intensive courses' took place three times a year, lasted for the inside of a week, and consisted partly of lectures and tutorials and partly of attendance at out-patient sessions. For each course there was a main theme – rheumatism, digestive complaints, gynaecological problems and so on.

Margery, when she became Dean, took these courses under her wing and transformed them. She had long anticipated that in the future, possibly in the near future, there would be a growing demand – an escalating demand – for homoeopathic treatment. And she was well aware that unless steps were taken at once there would be a grave shortage of qualified doctors who believed in homoeopathy and understood how to prescribe. It was therefore up to the Faculty to expand its teaching activities as much as possible. Obviously one could not expect to produce experts in five minutes, but one could make a start by enabling interested GPs to prescribe homoeopathic remedies intelligently on the National Health Service. The great gulf of misunderstanding between homoeopathy and medical-school medicine had to be bridged by personal contacts. To Margery this was axiomatic. The face-to-face encounter was her method in every context. Furthermore she anticipated that some of the GPs would be fired with enthusiasm and decide to train as full-time homoeopaths. It was part of her job to spot the likely ones. She was tireless in seeking out interested doctors. Before each course her handwritten notes of invitation, often scribbled in the car between London and Hedingham, went off in an unending stream, and with typical generosity she promised enticing subsidies: all expenses would be paid.★

When Margery took over the thrice-a-year courses she gave them a very special new flavour. Everything was imbued with her 'style'. Each course began early on a Monday morning and in the evening there was a 'fork supper' at Thurloe Street, a social occasion when new arrivals could become acquainted in very congenial surroundings, with wine and delicacies from Hedingham and flowers everywhere. The teaching sessions took place in Hahnemann House, adjoining the Royal London Homoeopathic Hospital, and on the Thursday evening there was a dinner at the Bedford Hotel in Bloomsbury (paid for by Margery out of her own pocket). This finale was planned so that the learners and the lecturers could mix in a friendly atmosphere.

★ Since Margery's death the financing of the courses has been reorganised, and participants now pay their own expenses.

These revitalised courses were such a success that some of the GPs came again and again. The first courses attracted a dozen or so, but after a few years the numbers were up to fifty, and eventually they reached more than a hundred. One of the young doctors concerned later gave a vivid account of how he came on an intensive course for the first time.

> I was working with a team of doctors in the Birmingham Eye Hospital and we were studying the toxic effects on the eye of modern drugs, and I got very fed up and thought, there must be an alternative. I got to know about homoeopathy and had some vague acquaintance with it. So I wrote to the Homoeopathic Hospital in London, expecting to get back some brochure, a typed notice of lectures or something, but no, I got a personal letter from Dr Blackie, and this amazed me. In it she explained that if I came, not only would I not have to pay, but my expenses would be paid, even those of a locum, and I thought 'What an amazing thing is this?'

He went on to describe his memories of Margery as a teacher. The experience of his first course affected him so deeply that he returned often.

> As I attended her lectures, I became aware of the differences in her lectures from any others I had ever heard. I was being caught up in a vision she had. I began to realize there was a fire burning down in Dr Blackie's heart and this was to make homoeopathy available to as many as possible.
>
> Her vision was to train doctors to this end, and the main theme that came over to us, as we listened to her, and were taught by her, was her absolute selflessness. She gave herself to us doctors whom she taught, nothing was too much trouble . . .
>
> While I listened to her lecturing I thought 'This is the lecturing, this is the teaching, I have always wanted to receive, this is real teaching'. She had this unique ability to be able to enthuse people with that same dedication and devotion – a real master.

'There are many doctors who for a long time will remember her lectures,' he concluded. 'As she described a remedy that remedy just lived, and you would come home and start to put it into practice. It was a wonderful experience to be taught by Dr Blackie.'

The gratitude of the GPs who came to Margery's courses must surely have meant much to her. One of them, Dorothy West, who later, for a time, worked at Thurloe Street as an assistant, wrote from her Devonshire practice after attending several courses:

> Once more I have felt the magic of one of your marvellous courses . . . Not only is the course exciting, stimulating and educational, it provides an atmosphere of such friendliness and warmth as one would find nowhere else. I feel sure this is entirely due to the very special spirit which you inject into it.
>
> I am having many successes here practising homoeopathy along the lines you have taught me.

During Margery's time as Dean of the Faculty, in 1971, the deaths occurred of two homoeopaths who were close to her, in very different ways. The first was Sir John Weir, who died in a nursing home in South London at the age of ninety-two. At the end the only doctor he would see was Margery, and she can hardly have failed to be moved by this – after so many years of rivalry.

But the second death was one which affected her much more deeply. The autumn of 1971 was a time of heartache and great sadness for her. Her faithful partner for more than forty years, Helena Banks, after suffering a long decline during which she had been forced by incurable gastric disabilities to give up her share in the practice, finally died on 4 October.

Letters of sympathy from patients poured in, and all paid tribute to Dr Banks's kindness. Some admitted that she had been 'straightforward and downright' and 'a watchdog' who protected Margery from intrusions, but all remembered her as exceptionally kind. There had been a saying:'If you are critically ill see Blackie; if you are convalescent see Banks.'

Margery had depended on 'Banks' in many ways and her death meant not only personal grief but dislocation in the practice. As a doctor she had always been ready to stand in for Margery when necessary and she had also kept the accounts, looked after the patients' records, taken charge of the telephone, acted as a welcoming receptionist, dealt with all the domestic arrangements, and in fact held the practice together as well as the household. When, gradually, she became unable to cope, and then later was confined to her room, suffering much pain, Musette came to London more often and began to take over as best she could. But things were not easy. She tried to keep the patients' records straight but was handicapped by lack of experience. One can imagine how poor Dr Banks must have felt, impotently bedridden upstairs. From the patients' viewpoint, too, the absence of Dr Banks was a sad loss. One lady who first consulted Margery at this time remembers that 'there was a fierce old woman in the hall, who ordered the patients about'. Nevertheless several others have insisted that if you could once get over Musette's gruff voice and unusual appearance you realised that she was a courteous and charming person.

For Margery herself it was a great support to have Musette at hand at a time when she was in distress for her dying friend, but eventually she decided to employ a professional secretary to deal with the business of the practice, and she found an efficient and devoted helper in Mrs Anne Barraclough, wife of Colonel Michael Barraclough, now Secretary to the Faculty of Homoeopathy.

As regards the medical aspect of the practice, during Dr Banks's last illness a new era had begun. Margery never took on another partner, but fully aware that she had to plan for the future, she adopted a policy of recruiting 'trainee assistants', mostly from among the younger doctors who had impressed her at the intensive courses. Her method was to let them sit in with her at her consultations for some months, and then in due course, when they were ready, they saw patients on their own. Writing to Frank Bodman in September 1967 she had said, 'There are three of us here, myself, Geoffrey Douch, and my new and most excellent assistant Anita Davies.' Dr Davies, who had first attended an intensive course two years previously, made rapid progress under Margery's training, and was soon helping her not only with patients at Thurloe Street but with the work of the Faculty. Another doctor who joined the team was an Australian, Max Deacon.

Meanwhile the intensive courses, which were introducing more and more GPs to 'The Principles and Practice of Homoeopathy' were for Margery an absorbing preoccupation, involving a mass of correspondence. Letter after letter, persuasive but firm, had to be sent to potential speakers. Some of them would need to make longish journeys to participate but in response to Margery's commands they came, Frank Bodman from Bristol, Alastair Jack from Birmingham, Frank Johnson from Newcastle, Alan Askew from Sheffield – these were her 'founder lecturers', her personal friends. She counted too on Anita Davies, at hand in London, and latterly also on a newcomer among her assistants, Charles Elliott, a talented and versatile Anglo-Irish doctor. Another regular lecturer was John Ainsworth, an experienced homoeopathic pharmacist, who explained, with the aid of a film, how the medicines were made.

Over the years Margery also roped in as speakers many homoeopathic doctors who were her professional acquaintances. These included Hamish Boyd, June Burger, Douglas Calcott, Donald Foubister, John Hughes-Games, Oliver Kennedy, Douglas MacKellar, Noel Pratt, Kathleen Priestman, John Raeside, Barry Rose, Stuart Semple, Dennis Somper and Ralph Twentyman. In addition she enlisted the help of a few speakers from outside homoeopathy, for instance Dr Richard Emanuel, the well-known cardiologist, with whom she was on warmly friendly terms.

Obviously the running of the intensive courses involved considerable expense, and although the Homoeopathic Research and Educational Trust gave some support, its financial help did not cover everything. Besides this, Margery found that dependence on the Trust was an irksome brake on her activity. Inevitably the strong aversion to bureaucracy that she shared with Musette asserted itself, and she was soon taking the situation in hand. Grateful patients often offered her generous gifts of money 'to help homoeopathy', and she and Musette decided to institute a fund, to be named the Blackie Foundation Trust, upon which she could call for finance as necessary. The initial capital of the Trust was £10,206, a sum largely derived from the proceeds of the Guildhall reception. Robin Holland-Martin, a patient of Margery's who worked in the City, was one of the three trustees, Margery and Musette the other two.

The objects of the Trust, which came into being in August 1971, were to be twofold; its capital and income were to be used for the teaching of homoeopathy, and money could also be made available for research. Henceforth Margery was able to manage things in the way she liked – a subsidy here, a subsidy there. Free from what she regarded as the 'interference' of committees, she could follow the biblical injunction 'Let not thy left hand know what thy right hand doeth'.

Catastrophe

Margery never flew. Her adamant prejudice against air travel was the main reason why she hardly ever went abroad, despite continual invitations; admirers and would-be patients had to come to London to see her. But it was also the reason why she escaped a terrible death in 1972, when a Trident airliner bound for Brussels crashed, with no survivors, shortly after take-off from Heathrow on Sunday 18 June. It was the worst air disaster in British history. A hundred and eighteen people were killed.

There was to be an International Homoeopathic Congress in Brussels the following week, and fifteen of the passengers – nine of them homoeopathic doctors – had been on their way to it. All were friends and acquaintances of Margery's. If she herself had been willing to fly she would almost certainly have been with them.

Overwhelmed by horror, shattered by grief, the world of homoeopathy mourned its dead, and the shared sorrow created a new bond between those who remained. The magnitude of the tragedy made the usual controversies and rivalries seem utterly petty. During a memorial service at the Church of St George the Martyr in Queen Square, close to the Royal London Homoeopathic Hospital, Dr Ralph Twentyman spoke with emotion of every one of the victims, and then went on to appeal for a new spirit of 'human purpose':

> Out of this, which feels like a stunning blow, there could, I believe, rise up a renewal, a renaissance, a rebirth of the human heart and human purpose and meaning in each one of us. Because

even our little world of medicine can never be – in the end – a matter of schools, a matter of science, a matter of some speciality. In the end it must be the care and concern and wisdom of doctor meeting patient, of one human person for another.

The weeks went by, and for a time the challenge to the homoeopathic community remained unforgettable. In the *British Homoeopathic Journal* the following verses were published.

AIR CRASH

The mind has lost credence.
The heart cannot encompass.
The will has no purpose.

So many of them –
part of our community body,
taken for granted,
sharing the everyday pattern –
now cut away.

They are so totally gone.
Not for them and for us
the gradual parting,
the gentler cutting of strands
one by one,
painful, yet accepted
at some level or other.

This is a clarion call
to the mind,
to the heart,
to the will.
Shocked to awareness,
we must find the focus,
fully awake now,
look at the pattern we make.

And those who have died
will be the seed
of the future.

For Margery a specially anguishing blow was the loss of a very promising young doctor who had recently become her protegé. Sergei William Kadleigh, known to his friends as 'Bill', had been an unusual person. Descended from Russian ancestry and belonging to the Orthodox Church, he had exceptional charm and what Margery called 'a real flair for homoeopathy'. 'He loved general practice and this is what he wanted to do,' she wrote after his death. 'He would indeed have been an expert homoeopathic physician.'

She had first met him when he came to one of the intensive courses, and she had found him immediately enthusiastic: 'he felt that homoeopathy was what he was looking for.' Subsequently he had come, at least once a week, sometimes oftener, to sit in at her practice, watching, learning. 'After finishing a hospital job he came into my practice as a full-time assistant and, as he said, he enjoyed every minute. We found him most congenial and cooperative to work with and the patients loved him. After only a month we received letters from dozens of patients telling of his sympathy and understanding.' Since his death, too, she added, his friends had been coming to ask about homoeopathy because 'Bill' had found it so inspiring and satisfying.

There was a further poignancy for Margery in Kadleigh's death. She had been quietly rejoicing to have found someone who might be worthy to serve as Physician to the Queen when the time came for her own retirement. And evidently she must have mentioned him to Her Majesty, for in a letter of condolence written in the Queen's own hand there is mention of him.

Thank you for your letter . . . I was extremely sorry to learn of the tragic death of nine doctors in the air crash at Staines, and I send my sincerest sympathy in this great loss to homoeopathy. To lose your own assistant must be a double blow and I do feel for you so much.

In addition to the trauma of bereavement there was a

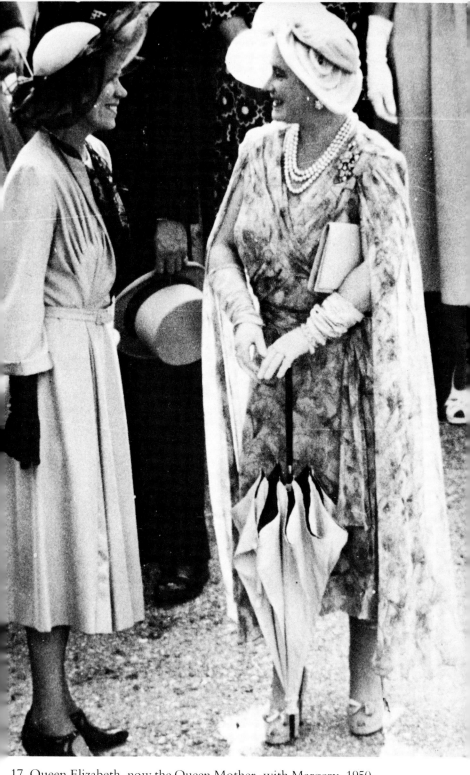

17 Queen Elizabeth, now the Queen Mother, with Margery, 1950

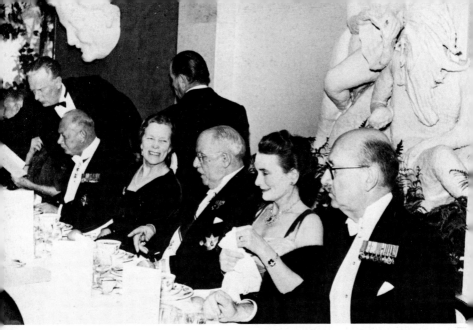

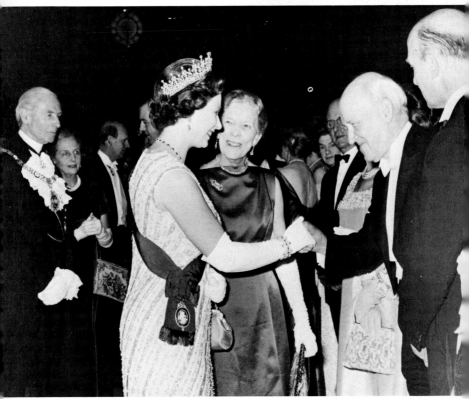

18 At a dinner for Sir John Weir; he sits between Princess Alice,
    Duchess of Gloucester, and Margery

19 At the 1970 Guildhall reception Dr Martyn Lloyd-Jones is
    presented to H.M. the Queen by Margery

repercussion from the Trident disaster which had far-reaching results that affected Margery in her work. One of the victims, Dudley Everitt, had long been a leading figure in homoeopathic pharmacy both in Britain and beyond, and he was the first such pharmacist to hold a Royal Warrant. His wife (who was killed with him in the crash) was a grand-daughter of the founder of London's best-known homoeopathic pharmacy, Nelson's in Duke Street, and for many years Everitt had been in charge of the family business. Under his direction Nelson's had maintained the highest reputation for excellence in dispensing.

After the Trident disaster the business had to be sold. The one surviving director, John Ainsworth, ran it for five years as Grantee of the Royal Warrants, but when the new owners carried out a reorganisation he left to set up his own pharmacy in New Cavendish Street. His wife, a cousin of Dudley Everitt's, became his co-director, and he had the support of pharmacist colleagues as well as active encouragement from Margery. His firm now holds the Royal Warrants to Her Majesty the Queen and to Her Majesty Queen Elizabeth the Queen Mother.

And what of Margery's state of mind as time went on after the disaster? Dr Charles Elliott has spoken of the amazing way in which she seemed to have overcome the shock, and he pays tribute to her resilience, determination, and fortitude. Even immediately after the memorial service at St George the Martyr, she had declared her resolve to 'keep on'. Her energy was phenomenal, he recalls, and it permeated life at Thurloe Street. Indeed he and her other assistants had to work under 'almost military discipline'. The routine was gruelling, especially on Mondays when the day started at six with 'Miss Majendie' out cleaning the car, and 'Aggie' getting breakfast at 6.30. 'Dr Blackie would be off to see patients at 7.45. There was never any morning break for coffee, and the "lunch hour" was only forty-five minutes. A glass of wine was allowed, but the phone was going all the time. Supper was at seven, and after it came the "planning phase", when post-graduate studies etc. were discussed till 9.30. Then the assistants left to go to bed, but Dr Blackie herself continued working till almost midnight' (on other weekday evenings there were often visits to patients after supper).

Meanwhile however the trauma of the Trident disaster took its toll of Margery's health. She was already in her seventies, and now, after bringing healing to countless patients she herself became a sufferer, stricken by acute rheumatoid arthritis in hands, wrists and knees. But with typical courage she steeled herself to 'keep on' and as much as possible concealed her affliction.

In the past her health had been very good on the whole. She 'did not have time to be ill'. When ailments occurred she knew what homoeopathic remedies to take, though doubtless, if she felt she needed a second opinion, she would have spoken with Helena Banks. But 'Banks' was no longer at hand. It was fortunate that she felt she could turn to her friend Alan Askew, a man of great sensitivity, upon whose judgement as a homoeopathic prescriber she knew she could rely. In her own words, 'No one ever carried out Hahnemann's teaching better.' He had started coming to Margery's intensive courses in his late forties, and had soon converted his Sheffield practice entirely to homoeopathy.

With the help of Askew's kindly expertise – he telephoned to her every day to check on her condition and to review his prescribing – Margery was able, to a remarkable extent, to get the better of her agonising disease. Although her walk was no longer brisk, as in earlier days, and her hands were too weak to pump up a blood-pressure machine, she was henceforth able to move her fingers without pain, to the great encouragement of her arthritic patients.

Margery regarded Askew as one of the rising stars of the younger generation of homoeopathic GPs, and was delighted that he lectured at her courses. She had also come to know him well off duty, because he often stayed briefly at Hedingham.

There he enlivened the scene, for he was a very likeable extrovert, a great all-round sportsman, with a special gift for caring for animals. He had many friends and they remember him, with a smile, as an 'original', a gastronome with a voracious appetite, who relished driving about in flashy cars.

After the Trident catastrophe Margery may well have felt that she had had her share of sudden bereavements. But a further shock was to come a few years later. In May 1977, during one of the intensive courses, when Askew had come to London to lecture, he died prematurely, suddenly, from a heart attack.

During the decade that followed the Trident disaster the term 'alternative medicine' gradually became a household word. And in common usage it began to include all the various therapies which differ from the medical-school medicine of today – not only homoeopathy but acupuncture, osteopathy, chiroprac, herbalism, radionics ('the black box') and so on. In Margery's view however there was only one 'alternative' that really mattered, the classical homoeopathy, as taught by Hahnemann, that she so faithfully practised and that she fervently believed should be defended against corruption.

It was therefore with grave apprehension that during the 1970s, as Dean of the Faculty of Homoeopathy, she witnessed an accelerating swing away from Hahnemann towards Rudolf Steiner. Quite a number of her colleagues shared her dismay, notably her friend from resident days, Frank Bodman, while her fellow-Christian homoeopaths were especially disturbed: Alastair Jack, a dedicated Christian whom she termed a *real* homoeopathic GP, Frank Johnson, another clear-sighted Christian, and Anita Davies, her chief assistant at Thurloe Street, who had attended the Westminster Chapel from her student days, before ever she met Margery.

Matters came to a head in 1974, with a controversy about the editorial policy of the *British Homoeopathic Journal*. Pride of place was being given to articles connected with Steiner's teachings. Three issues had been conspicuously dominated by instalments of a study in 'neo-astrology' entitled 'The Signature of the Planet Mercury in Plants'. In meticulous detail it dealt with the effect of constellations on plant saps, and its purpose was to identify the most favourable days for gathering the mistletoe required to produce *Iscador*, the anthroposophical preparation for the treatment of cancer. In Margery's eyes the implication that homoeopathy could be identified with the occult was entirely unacceptable, and she had noticed that classical homoeopaths were withholding their articles. She confided her anxiety to Frank Bodman: 'I am in despair about the journal,' she wrote. 'Most people don't want their cases put in between anthroposophy and don't send. I find there is a great reluctance to send things in.' Furthermore she felt that the journal's bias gave an utterly wrong impression of what homoeopathy *is*, an impression which would undoubtedly be seriously off-putting to any doctors or medical students who might come across copies of the journal in the libraries of the teaching hospitals up and down the country. Bodman agreed with her whole-heartedly, and also pointed out that there had been pronouncements in the journal dismissing classical homoeopathy as an inadequate guide to prescribing, which only led to confusion in the minds of new recruits.

Another cause for alarm, so Margery felt, was the infiltration of non-classical treatments in the London hospital. Many of the patients did not get homoeopathy at all, which was seriously disquieting to the younger doctors. Trouble had also been brewing in connection with the intensive courses, and a little later Margery wrote emphatically to Alastair Jack, 'We must have basic homoeopathy taught and not Rudolf Steiner philosophy.'

In all these ways, for Margery and for those who agreed with her, the outlook seemed dark indeed.★

★ Since Margery's death the Faculty has continued to include anthroposophists as well as supporters of classical homoeopathy. But in the journal there are now fewer articles by anthroposophists than previously.

But meanwhile, outside London, a new era was dawning. Throughout Britain there were regional branches of the Faculty, and in Birmingham, where Alastair Jack headed the Midlands Branch, a series of yearly one-day symposia for interested GPs was being launched at the Post-Graduate Centre of the Selly Oak Hospital. Dr Jack and other experienced homoeopaths were also to follow up with half-day tutorials, and nothing but the classical version was to be taught. Anthroposophical medicine would *not* be an optional alternative.

In the autumn of 1975 Margery was invited to speak at the first of these symposia. She had only just recovered from her rheumatoid arthritis but she did manage to make the journey, accompanied by Musette, who had also been ill. 'We have had rather a poor two years on the whole,' she wrote to Dr Jack, 'but I am well, and she is getting well so we feel cheered.' Then, as though to prove that she was really herself again, she added, 'I still carry on one surgery a week here and get a wonderful cross-section of illnesses and types.'

That first Birmingham symposium, attended by seventy-five doctors, more than half of them new to homoeopathy, kindled new hope in Margery's heart; here was a positive means for maintaining the highest standards in the future. Immediately after it she sent Dr Jack a generous donation from the Blackie Foundation Trust for his Midlands Branch. 'I feel very encouraged by the response in Birmingham,' she told him. 'Perhaps that will be the first place to have a regular clinic, but I'm sure you're right to start with the interested doctors as you're doing. And I'm so thankful to be able to help from the Foundation Trust. It's what I always meant it for.' In the following year she went again to Birmingham for the autumn symposium, and afterwards wrote to say it had been 'a real inspiration'.

The gatherings of the Midlands Branch, which were soon attracting up to a hundred GPs, now became an annual event in her life. And meanwhile little scribbled notes – 'I believe you'll be running short of funds . . .' – were frequently dispatched from Thurloe Street, accompanied by cheques ranging from £100 to £300. 'I am thrilled with all you do in the Midlands Branch,' she wrote. 'It has been one of my very greatest pleasures to be able to contribute to your great effort.'

During her visits to Birmingham Margery also became interested in a further development. Dr Jack had realised – as Margery herself had of late come to admit – that if the critics and opponents of homoeopathy were ever to be convinced, 'proof' of the therapy would have to be given in scientific terms. Clinical evidence alone would never suffice. This view was fully shared by another Birmingham enthusiast, Dr Robin Pinsent, who was Research Adviser to the Royal College of General Practitioners. Thanks to Dr Pinsent's initiative an interdisciplinary research group was formed 'to encourage and conduct rigorous objective examination of the principles and practice of homoeopathy'. Margery herself agreed to be Honorary Consultant Adviser to the new group, which at its formation included a professor of pharmacology, an academic metallurgist, a psychiatrist, a consulting physician and also a number of GPs. When word got round about this research, many experienced homoeopaths in all parts of the British Isles became working members of the group, and in 1977 it attained formal status as the Midlands Homoeopathy Research Group.

Margery's main reasons for her opposition to anthroposophy were firstly that she regarded it as anti-Christian, and secondly that in her view – her very practical view – it was 'woolly-minded'. But she was not prejudiced against every alternative therapy other than her own. Some of them, indeed, she recommended to her patients on occasion. 'She was not exclusive,' one of her friends has insisted. 'She brought in anything that could do good. For her, healing was the all-important thing.'

In the case of acupuncture, which she herself had studied, she maintained that it could be practised without accepting the philosophy behind it. And one of the letters of congratulation she received at the time of her royal appointment shows that she put this belief into practice. A former patient wrote to her, 'I cannot possibly expect you to remember me, but I have always appreciated your kindness and help when I received acupuncture treatment at the Homoeopathic Hospital about four years ago.'

A letter from another patient is evidence that manipulation, too, was a method she sometimes found appropriate. The writer told her that as a child she used to visit her surgery with her mother: 'You were always very kind to me and cured me of all aches and pains by manipulating the bones in my neck and back by stretching, pulling, and so forth.'

Osteopathy was yet another therapy which Margery sometimes recommended, but she drew the line, very definitely, at radionics. When in her earlier days she had supported William Boyd and his Glasgow research into physical dynamics, and had derived help in diagnosis from his Emanometer, she had not given much thought to the principles involved. But the more recent developments in radionics and radiasthesia, identifying them as forms of extra-sensory perception, along with clairvoyance and other paranormal phenomena, caused her to shrink back. She did not wish to be involved in exploring or making use of therapies which she regarded as verging on the occult. Her terse comment on the 'black box' was 'black magic!'

Apologia

'I have been so terribly hard worked since my book came out,' Margery wrote joyfully to Alastair Jack in July 1976. 'I have had three hundred letters in one week, mostly asking for appointments.' Her book *The Patient, Not the Cure* was her final apologia, her great summing up of the cause to which she had devoted her life. In it she had attempted to encompass many diverse aspects of homoeopathy. There were chapters on Hahnemann, on his discoveries and teachings, on the leading homoeopaths since his time, on the remedies and their preparation, on the methods of the practitioner. There was also a chapter on 'the contemporary scene'. She refrained from mentioning the conflict within the Faculty, but several times insisted that 'homoeopathy is not a philosophy: it is a science based on observation and experience'.

The idea that Margery should write such a book had originated with the publishers Macdonald & Jane, who saw an urgent need for a work on homoeopathy 'suitable for really interested laymen'.

At first Margery said she could not possibly undertake the task, but in the end they persuaded her, and for about eighteen months she 'made the time', helped indispensably by a number of friends. It was an amazing achievement to produce the book at all when she was already so busy, but perhaps inevitably the result resembles a fine piece of patchwork rather than an integrated work of art.

As to the publisher's aim – to cater for really interested laymen – much of the book meets this requirement, and it provides valuable definitions, in simple language, of homoeopathy's basic tenets. For example, in the introduction, Margery wrote: 'Throughout the history of medicine there is a tendency to treat diseases by methods which were applied to people en masse. Hahnemann's homoeopathic principle is to treat the individual in order to bring the whole man back to his true state of health.'

It must be admitted however that some sections of the book abound in technical terms, and are therefore more suited to medical students than to the uninitiated. Nevertheless a great deal of interest was aroused. During the first two weeks after publication the staff of the British Homoeopathic Association (a society aimed at spreading the knowledge and use of homoeopathy among the laity) had to deal with as many as seventeen hundred letters. More recently, furthermore, it has held its own. There have been two reprints, and a paperback edition (published by Unwin) is currently available under the title *The Challenge of Homoeopathy*.

Like all Margery's writings *The Patient, Not the Cure* was made up largely of case histories, or rather anecdotes.* And this meant, as Frank Bodman pointed out in his review for the *British Homoeopathic Journal*, that it would surely be anathema to the medical establishment, which regards 'anecdote' as a dirty word because it is anti-statistical. But, so he went on to explain in Margery's defence, results in homoeopathic practice can hardly be described at all without resorting to anecdote. 'Individuals of necessity vary so much that they do not lend themselves to statistical treatment . . . patients with the same diagnostic label require different medicines.'

It was only to be expected that reviews in homoeopathic publications would be appreciative, but not all the 'outsiders' who took notice of the book were unsympathetic. The *New*

---

* Some of these, in the chapter 'Homoeopathy on the Farm', showed how cattle, dogs, fowls and especially horses could be helped by the right remedies. Margery had had personal experience of prescribing for horses belonging to some of her VIP patients.

Scientist reviewer, for one, took an objective attitude. 'Homoeopathy is unique among the systems of alternative medicine,' he wrote, 'for its headquarters in Britain is the Royal London Homoeopathic Hospital, an institution belonging to the NHS.'

> Dr Blackie is the senior and most renowned of the physicians practising Hahnemann's ideas today . . . Her methods and beliefs . . . may well provoke scorn and derision, or at least condescending smiles, among her more orthodox colleagues in the medical trade, but even the most proficient and successful medical technologists would do well to ponder on an approach to healing which, however irrational, clearly brings comfort and relief to many who are sick.

Still there was plenty of 'scorn and derision' elsewhere, although the book evidently gave pause to even the most outspoken critics. The review in *Medical News* was headed 'Homoeopathy: Art, Science or Paramedical Delusion?'. But it ended with a frank admission: 'Few doctors are so satisfied with what conventional treatment has to offer as to neglect alternative approaches altogether . . . It is a book to make us stop and think.'

Even the *British Medical Journal*, which started with a scathing swipe, went on to some second thoughts. 'This book will be a universal success,' the review began. 'Homoeopaths will be filled with pride that what they have always believed is right, and allopaths [non-homoeopathic doctors] will be delighted that they have never had any truck with all this rubbish. The book makes it quite clear what rubbish homoeopathy is intellectually.' But then the tone changed:

> It would be as well for the materialistic, or empirical, scientist to realise that not all the world believes in scientific proof, or . . . rather that science ought to concern itself only with what is for the good of mankind.
>
> Most sensible people would agree that homoeopathy is . . . better than the overprescription of modern powerful and dangerous drugs and mountains of tranquillisers, in all but the few cases

of serious organic disease. The bulk of ordinary practice consists
of neurotic disorders . . . and homoeopathic attention to the
patient and her symptoms are more acceptable than our attention
to the machines and the laboratory. Not all doctors listen enough,
or take enough time, with undiagnosable ailments.

Yet in spite of this concession, the reviewer still claimed that
there are unarguable grounds for rejecting homoeopathy. The
basic difficulty about it, he asserted, and an insuperable one, 'is
that it claims an exclusive system of belief'.

How wrong he was! At least in the case of Margery Blackie.
For although she was unwaveringly faithful to classical
homoeopathic principles, she never denied that there were
cases where other therapies and treatments were necessary. It
goes without saying that for her the supreme precedent for
co-operation with doctors who were not homoeopaths was
her harmonious relationship with her fellow physicians in the
Royal Medical Household. But in addition to this she had
cordial connections with many of the leading London specialists, and at the clinical level she co-operated with pathologists,
gynaecologists, rheumatologists, orthopaedic surgeons,
neurologists and others. By all of these she was held in high
esteem, and if she advised a patient to consult one of them she
made a point of going along to the consultation.

In an interview with an Australian journalist just after her
book was published (when she revealed the interesting information that she had an estimated seven thousand patients in
her practice) she was questioned on this very point, as to
whether she found that homoeopathy could be combined with
non-homoeopathic medicine, and she replied that she had no
hesitation in advising a patient to seek the opinion of a
specialist if the case warranted it. 'I may ask a specialist to treat
a particular patient I have seen or, in a case where surgery is
indicated, I may treat the patient before and after operation. In
some cases homoeopathic treatment may make surgery un-
necessary.'

In this connection it is interesting to recall an incident which

remains vividly in the memory of one of Margery's colleagues, Dr Frank Johnson, especially as it shows up several of
her characteristic traits – her quick reactions, her tendency to
anger, and her ability to apologise humbly. Dr Johnson used
to come to London from the north of England to take part in
her intensive courses, and at one of these, after she had been
speaking, someone asked, 'Dr Blackie, what do you give for
appendicitis?' Immediately came the crisp reply, 'I'd give
Colchicum.'* This spurred Dr Johnson to spring to his feet and
exclaim, 'Surely Dr Blackie means that she would call a surgeon
and then give *Colchicum* while awaiting him.' Margery had of
course meant precisely that, but she had slipped up in her
answer: even so she was deeply offended. She was not accustomed to being contradicted in public and she would not speak
to Johnson for quite a time. Eventually she wrote to him: 'I
have waited to write to you until my annoyance subsided, and
I would now beg of you not to behave again as you did.' To
this he wrote back: 'I was shocked at the tenor and wording of
your letter. If your reference to my behaviour refers to the
lecture which touched upon the treatment of diagnosed appendicitis I have no apologies to make . . . I therefore, with
regret, withdraw from the London scene.' Perhaps she had
not expected such a strong reaction, for she hastened to write
again: 'Please forget my letter and come back to lecture. I can't
do without you . . . and I apologise for offending you . . .
Send me a line to Hedingham to put my mind at rest.'

The Patient, Not the Cure is prefaced by a dedication and a
paragraph of acknowledgements, both of which reflect
Margery's closest personal relationships. She dedicated the
book to 'The late Dr Helena F. Banks, my friend and partner
of over thirty years', and in the acknowledgments she wrote:
'My deep gratitude is due to my friend Musette Majendie,
CBE, for her constant helpfulness and advice during the
writing of this book'.

* A homoeopathic remedy derived from meadow saffron.

As to her colleagues, she made grateful mention of Frank
Bodman, Anita Davies, Alan Askew, Alastair Jack and John
Ainsworth. But first on the list of those who had given her
help – ahead of all the others – was Dr Martyn Lloyd-Jones, to
whom she expressed her grateful thanks 'for his kindness in
sparing the time to read the proofs'. In fact he had done a great
deal more. Margery had turned to him again and again while
working on the book. They spoke on the telephone almost
every day. And his wife Bethan, herself a doctor, also made
valuable comments.

But of course Margery's association with Dr Lloyd-Jones
was not only on the level of literary advice. As she grew older
she was relying more and more on him as her spiritual guide.
In the past she had been chiefly influenced, like so many
others, by his preaching, those penetrating expositions of the
Christian faith which had drawn thousands to the Westminster Chapel. Now, since his retirement in 1968, his pastoral care
for her took the form of private talks. There were opportunities for these when he and his wife visited Hedingham.

Meanwhile he, on his side, had come to rely on Margery as a
physician. Although he never became a devotee of
homoeopathy in the exclusive sense, he found many of the
homoeopathic medicines efficacious, and was happy to use
them, both for himself and his family. Thus Margery helped
him with timely prescriptions, and also with welcoming
hospitality at Hedingham; he convalesced there after his first
cancer operation.

And for her, friendship with the great preacher brought a
further blessing, the chance to be in touch with an inspiring
example of a disciplined life – a life of prayer, worship and
trust in God. Although she was by nature courageous there
were times when her courage was put to the test. Once at
Thurloe Street the small lift to the upper floors broke down,
and Margery, who was alone in it, was trapped in the dark. Far
from panicking she spent the time until she was rescued
singing hymns. She had a lovely singing voice.

Retirement

Margery remained the 'First Lady' of homoeopathy until the very end, looked up to with heartfelt gratitude and affection by thousands of patients, as well as by the scores of doctors who had learnt from her. And among her fellow homoeopaths, even those who disagreed with her acknowledged that as a leader, over many long years, she had been far and away ahead of them all.

Yet inevitably, as she passed her eightieth birthday, there were signs which could not be ignored that she was beginning to wear out. Her memory – her wonderful memory – often let her down now, and this was a serious matter. Hitherto at consultations she had seldom referred to written notes, and her letters were always in longhand, so there were no carbon copies for reference. She was also slightly deaf and had to make use of a hearing aid and an amplifying telephone. Meantime her dynamic vitality and her firm grasp as a planner were flagging. In the past she had relished the hard work of running the intensive courses, and had found the controversies within the Faculty a stimulus. But now no longer. Although sometimes she was her 'old self', at other times she was certainly not. One of her friends, grieved to see these changes in her, has called this last stage of her life 'a nebulous time'.

In the autumn of 1978 Alastair Jack was deeply concerned to see how exhausted she was after the October intensive courses, and he wrote her a long and understanding letter, begging her to ease up. He often asked himself, he said, why Alan Askew's second coronary came when it did. 'Was it because of the extra strain he encountered at the course? I am selfish enough not to want to lose you prematurely.' With great tact he also raised the question of whether the time had come for her to resign as Dean of the Faculty. He urged her to stay on but insisted that somehow she must find a way of delegating most of her responsibility. Even as he wrote, however, he must have known very well that it was not in Margery's nature to delegate. In late November, after she had taken part for the last time in a Birmingham symposium (she came by car from Hedingham, there and back in a day, a round trip of 350 miles) Musette telephoned to him to say that the decision had been made. Margery was going to resign as Dean at the end of the academic year.

For fifteen years she had held the reins, and her teaching, along with her work for her patients, had been what she cared about most in her professional life. Thus when she announced, at a Council meeting in February 1979, that she would not seek re-election, it was a solemn moment. And not only for herself. A few of her colleagues had already been hinting openly that her time was up, but when she actually announced that she was leaving they were all of them shaken. 'The dignity of the occasion was somewhat overwhelming,' Dr June Burger wrote to her afterwards. 'Your enthusiasm has always been an inspiration. No doubt there will be changes, but what you have brought, out of your own enthusiasm and personality, will not be matched.' These last two remarks were very true. After Margery stood down changes did indeed take place. But her unique contribution to the homoeopathic cause has been acknowledged ever since. And the memory of all she had done has been kept visibly alive: a portrait of her, painted by James Gunn, hangs in the boardroom of the Royal London Homoeopathic Hospital where Faculty meetings are held. There she sits, ageless and erect, in a simple wine-coloured velvet gown, looking down on the changing scene with a flicker of an enigmatic smile on her lips, alongside Hahnemann, Quin, Clarke and Weir.

In several ways 1979 was a critical year for homoeopathy in Britain. During the spring and summer Margery was heavily involved in politics in an attempt to save the Royal London Homoeopathic Hospital, which under the National Health Service seemed to be doomed to closure. Her interest in the hospital was not only for the sake of the patients. 'It is the centre of homoeopathic teaching in this country,' she declared, 'and must be kept so.' Interviewed by the *Evening News*, just before a petition with 36,500 signatures was to be presented to a mass lobby of MPs, she asserted that she was confident the hospital would stay open. So it did, but only on a declining scale. For despite the efforts of the great supporter of homoeopathy in Parliament, Mr Tom Ellis, MP for Wrexham, and despite a further petition with 116,781 signatures which was presented in the House of Commons in July, the relentless bureaucratic 'streamlining' of the NHS continued undeterred. In September 1979 the Camden and Islington Area Health Authority was told to cut £2 million off its expenditure and the Authority picked on the Homoeopathic Hospital as not needed by the local people and therefore the first to be 'reorganised'. Since then, little by little, various wards have been closed, and the number of beds available for homoeopathic medicine is now less than a third what it was in the hospital's heyday. The out-patient department has remained flourishing, but the name 'Royal London Homoeopathic Hospital', which proudly decorates the front of the main building, is a fading reminder of its former glory.★

During 1979, Margery's eighty-second year, she felt obliged to give up several commitments which meant much to her, in

★ Early in 1984, the Bloomsbury Health Authority announced a plan to create a main centre for complementary medicine within the hospital building, to include acupuncture, osteopathy, chiropractic and manipulative medicine. For homoeopathic medicine 44 beds were to be retained and the out-patient facilities were to be expanded.

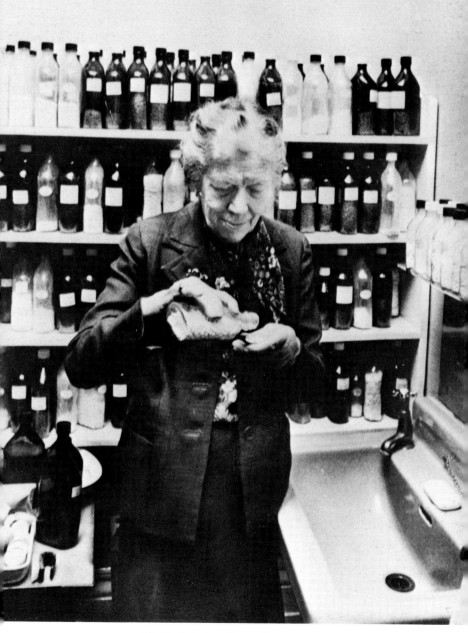

20 Dr Blackie dispensing

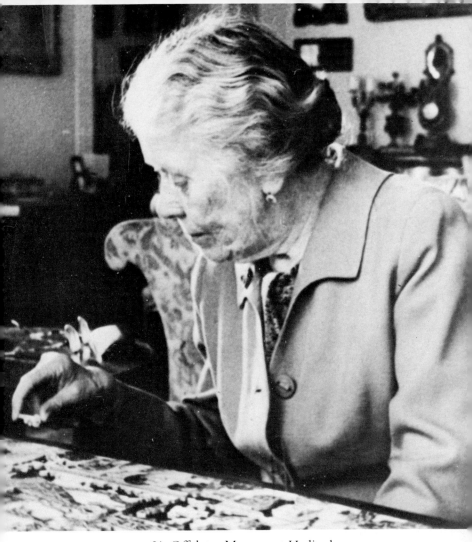

21 Off duty: Margery at Hedingham

addition to the Deanship. Foremost of these, of course, was her position as a member of the Royal Medical Household, a position of trust that she had held for a decade with the utmost integrity. 'She was very discreet,' one of her fellow homoeo-paths has said, 'never revealing any confidences about her most illustrious patients, even to her closest colleagues.'

A further tribute to her service has been made by Sir Richard Bayliss, who from 1973 was Head of the Royal Medical Household. It is a significant tribute, for it throws light upon Margery's attitude towards non-homoeopathic medicine. When Sir Richard was asked recently for his memories of working with Margery, he replied with enthusiasm, 'She was a great doctor. She had amazing intuition and her mind was sharp as a whiplash. She was *marvellous* to work with. We *never* had a disagreement. She never asked me not to prescribe such and such a drug. After all, she herself had had a full training in general medicine.' To illustrate her judgement he recalled an occasion when the Queen Mother, who held Margery in warmly affectionate regard, and always called her in first if she needed medical help, was laid low with bronchi-tis. After a day or so Margery telephoned to Bayliss and said, 'I think she is going to need penicillin.'*

Margery's devoted service to the royal family was given formal recognition in the 1979 New Year's Honours, when she was appointed to the Royal Victorian Order in the rank of Commander, and then in June came her resignation. 'That splendid lady Dr Margery Blackie has quietly retired as the Queen's homoeopathic doctor,' announced the *Evening News*, under the headline 'Queen's Fringe Doctor bows out'.

It was in that same year, 1979, that Margery very reluctantly withdrew from the intensive courses. She was due to speak at

---

* Sir Richard's confidence in Margery was fully reciprocated. She often advised her patients to consult him, and a few years before her retirement, in 1975, she had turned to him on behalf of Musette, who was suffering from hyperthyroid trouble. He was able to treat her successfully, and he remem-bers Margery saying to him, 'There was nothing *I* could have done for her.'

the May course but did not appear, and for the October course
she was not billed. Nor was she able to attend the autumn
symposium of the Midlands Group in Birmingham. In October she wrote to Alastair Jack: 'Would you mind if Musette
and I don't come. We'd love to and I have prepared a talk, but
we are both a bit poor . . . How terribly sad we are and I hate
to miss that lovely day.' Yet in spite of the decline in her
abilities her enthusiasm for the symposia at Birmingham did
not slacken, and by means of the Blackie Foundation Trust she
continued her financial support.

At this time there was a development which was soon to
have important results for the research activities in Birmingham. Through Margery's connection with Dr Martyn Lloyd-
Jones and the Westminster Chapel she was introduced to a
doctor named Ronald Davey, a committed Christian. Dr
Davey's special interest was in bringing his scientific medical
training to bear upon the question 'How does homoeopathy
work?' and largely thanks to him a research division of the
Blackie Foundation Trust was later formed.* This division
was soon to be co-ordinated with the Midlands Homoeopathy
Research Group, and latterly the joint organisation became the
British Homoeopathy Research Group, with a base in London.

In the spring of 1979 there was a very successful occasion in
aid of the Blackie Foundation Trust, the last of its kind at
which Margery was present. A patient of hers, Mrs Lillian
Sheepshanks, who lived in Suffolk, was so rapturously grateful for the recovery of her son, who under Margery's care had
overcome a particularly distressing bone disease, that she was
inspired to organise a special fund-raising concert as a gesture
of thanks. The event took place at Aldeburgh in the Maltings
Concert Hall at Snape, and it consisted of music, reading and
recitations. All the performers, including Dame Wendy
Hiller, Thomas Hemsley the baritone and Peter Pears the

---

* After Margery's death Dr Davey took on the responsibility of directing
both the educational and the research activities of the Trust.

tenor, were people who had reason to be thankful for homoeopathy.

For Margery the Snape concert was a severe challenge, since only a short time before it she had fallen and fractured a hip. But undaunted as ever she insisted on being there, elegant even in a wheelchair, to greet her royal patient who had become her dear friend, Queen Elizabeth the Queen Mother.

After her accident Margery was unable to walk for quite a time, and she found the enforced inactivity very trying. However she managed to get to her feet again and went on seeing patients at Thurloe Street. This meant that even now she could continue her teaching work. For with the patients' permission she still admitted other doctors as observers to some of her consultations. One of them has said, 'It was a privilege to see the medical consultation at its best.'

Margery finally left London for good in the spring of 1980. She did not arrange for the practice to be taken over, but 18 Thurloe Street, which had been left by Dr Banks to a nephew and niece, was sold in such a way that a continuing association with homoeopathy was ensured (it is now a centre for homoeopathy and alternative medicine). While the sale was being negotiated Margery's patients still came as usual to number 18, where Anita Davies took charge. Subsequently they were able to choose which of the doctors who had been Margery's pupils they wished to go to. Some patients who lived outside London decided to consult doctors who practised nearer their homes; Margery had encouraged the opening of homoeopathic clinics in places such as Chichester (Max Deacon) and Winchester (Trevor Smith).

In the meantime Charles Elliott succeeded Margery in her supreme responsibility. He had been introduced to Her Majesty the Queen by Margery herself, and in due course he was appointed to the Royal Medical Household, with the position that Margery had held before him.

The last year and a half of Margery's life, the final stage of her retirement, was spent at Hedingham, which was now her only home, and where Musette was like an only sister to her. An only sister? What about Kay Blackie and Lillian Townend? Margery did not cut herself off from the surviving members of her family, but she firmly discouraged their efforts to share in her life. Kay, who died in 1978, and Lillian had for some years been coming to stay at Hedingham at Christmas and Easter. But Margery had not looked forward to their visits, for her elder sisters expected to have everything their own way, and did not hesitate to say so. This was upsetting to Musette as well as to Margery, and when Lillian, and also Margery's brother Frank, showed that they would like to settle near Hedingham, both Margery and Musette drew the line. It would never have worked.

Musette, although she was younger than Margery, protected her from her family. She also sheltered Margery from realising how ill she was, and from dwelling upon the prospect of death. Musette would not admit, even to herself, that her beloved friend would never be 'the same' again. During the last period of Margery's life her mind sometimes wandered, and Musette was constantly on the watch so as to save her from embarrassment.

But Musette's own health was failing. After a slight stroke she tried to keep going as usual, but before long her condition could not be concealed, and in the end it became necessary to have day and night nurses. She died of a heart attack on 24 January 1981. For Margery this shattering bereavement was soon followed by another. Dr Martyn Lloyd-Jones, whose cancer had long been held at bay, finally died on 1 March.

Without Musette the ménage at Hedingham could not continue, even though for several years the running of it had been under the direction of a very efficient 'lady administrator', Mrs Joyce Westmorland. During the early months of 1981 the residents made plans to leave. They were all of them elderly men and women who had been sharing life together for quite a time, mostly widows and widowers. Lady Lascelles, a long-time friend of both Musette and Margery,

had been at Hedingham since the death of her husband Sir
Francis Lascelles, formerly Clerk of the Parliaments. Myles
Routledge, a genial Old Harrovian, had been a resident since
the loss of his second wife. There was also one married couple,
a retired Vice-Provost of Eton, Julian Lambart, and his wife.
For Margery as well as for the residents themselves, the enforced break-up of the little community of kindred spirits was
a tragedy.

After the residents had dispersed the great house was a
depressingly empty place. Fortunately however Joyce Westmorland took charge of the situation. During her time at
Hedingham she had become a devoted friend and companion
to Margery (as well as to Musette) and she understood her
very well. She had been living nearby at the Garden House,
the 'cottage' which had formerly been lent to Dr Banks, and at
the end of May she arranged to take Margery there, so that she
could look after her more easily, in a cosier atmosphere. She
did indeed look after her, hand and foot, unstintingly, and
thanks to her dedicated care Margery was cherished lovingly
during her last three months.

As regards homoeopathic treatment at this time, Margery
was attended by three of her closest colleagues, Charles
Elliott, Alastair Jack and Frank Johnson. Dr Johnson came
from the north of England to prescribe for her, and he
remembers that at first he jibbed at the distance involved. But
Margery insisted, and 'when Margery insisted there was no
questioning'.

During the summer months of 1981 Margery became increasingly frail, and although she understood all that was
going on she spoke very little. Her love of birds was still a joy
to her, however, and she would spend hours watching them
hopping about on a special bird table outside the window.
Occasionally, too, she was wheeled out to sit in the garden,
dressed as usual in one of her Lachasse outfits. And sometimes
Joyce took her for drives. She liked looking out at places she
knew, and specially noticed the churches. She was no longer

able to attend church services, but a retired Anglican clergy-man brought Holy Communion to her at the Garden House and this meant much to her.

There were two books always at her bedside, her homoeopathic 'bible', Kent's *Materia Medica*, and the Bible itself. She had always loved the Book of Deuteronomy, as had also Musette, and towards the end, when she herself was unable to read, she often asked Joyce to read aloud from it.

Margery died peacefully on 24 August 1981 after a stroke, and her funeral took place five days later at the Castle Hedingham parish church. She was buried next to her dearest friend, Musette Majendie. Later, in London, at the Church of St James in Piccadilly, there was a memorial service. A packed congregation listened as the service began with a bidding spoken by one of Margery's clergy friends, David Maddock, formerly Suffragan Bishop of Dunwich. He had greatly admired and loved Margery and he brought out, in moving terms, that not only had she fulfilled her vocation as an inspired healer during her life on earth, but henceforth she would be continuing her service to God.

We meet to give thanks to God for the privilege of having known Margery Blackie. Here we shall see her no more, but we believe that God still has work for her to do:

My body is the sheath,
My spirit is the sword.
God draws the sword for His own use.
Men call it death.

As we remember her we give thanks for her intellectual eminence, her healing skill, her courage, her charm, her humanity, her joyous gift of friendship, but above all for her love of God, from which all these graces spring. The essence of sanctity is dedication, and it is of her dedication to God and to the work which she knew He had called her to do, her calling, her vocation, that we think as we associate her with all the saints.

Achievement

The powerful influence of Margery Blackie, of her example and her teaching, lives on in the doctors who learnt their homoeopathy from her. One has only to mention her name and eyes light up. Why was she so inspiring? What was her impetus? And what were the characteristics of the homoeopathy that she taught with such a lasting impact?

In the first place, the driving force behind everything she taught and did as a physician was the belief she summed up in the title of her book *The Patient, Not the Cure*. The healing of the individual patient, the 'making whole' of the sick man, woman or child, was her essential, overriding purpose. She did not rule out the usefulness of homoeopathic 'first aid' – it was good that common ailments could be alleviated by remedies bought over the counter. But the homoeopathy at which she excelled so notably was the treatment of long-term chronic diseases – 'heart trouble', high blood pressure, the rheumatisms, skin affections, allergies, and all the rest.

Her homoeopathy was primarily concerned with finding the one medicine that was appropriate for a particular patient. She did not seek to achieve 'instant cures', but rather to restore the patient's interior balance. Long before the currently fashionable term 'the holistic approach' was coined, Margery was a spontaneous master of the art.

Each patient was for her unique. To Margery there was no such thing as 'a case of hay fever'. There was Tom's hay fever, Dick's hay fever, Harry's hay fever. To her there was no such thing as 'a case of arthritis', there was Mary's arthritis, Anne's arthritis, Joan's arthritis. She believed that in each unique person, before the symptoms had become manifest, there had been some kind of interior upset, and her aim was to restore the equilibrium of mind and body. She knew that the affected part – if the structure had not been damaged beyond repair – would then again take on its normal function. This process sometimes demanded great patience, and occasionally it was necessary to prescribe a series of remedies over long periods. But perhaps Margery's greatest gift was for high-potency prescribing, which in her skilled hands brought immediate response.

Obviously her methods were in direct contrast to the methods of much contemporary medicine, which aim at suppressing every pain and troublesome symptom, meanwhile accepting the likelihood of side-effects and the prospect of possibly adverse repercussions in the future.

Margery's attitude to apparently intractable disease was also the antithesis of the current norm. She refused to accept the well-worn saying 'You'll have to live with it'. Innumerable patients who had been given up by their doctors, and told they had to live with it, found hope and healing under her care – under her application of 'the gentle art'. 'In Dr Blackie's consulting room', a medical journalist once wrote, 'you will see the medical rubbish dump . . . the cases that nobody, not even the Big Boss, can do anything for.'

'Difficult' patients were treated by her with the same kindness and patience as all the others. And this was no mere sentimentality. Margery knew what she was doing. In one of her presidential addresses she quoted the saying that nine-tenths of the difficult patients are difficult because their doctors have been unable or unwilling to appreciate their fears or peculiar problems. 'Unless the doctor is utterly devoted to his patients, and prepared to take immense trouble to understand their problems, he is inferior to a machine.' Compassion was her touchstone. And she was well aware that in the medical profession today there is often, alas, little time for it.

Margery has been accused of practising in a backwater, of ignoring the meteoric advances of modern medicine. This is an entirely unjust charge. She saw clearly what was happening in the world of medicine, and she often guided her patients towards non-homoeopathic treatment. But she also saw the price that was being paid for many of the 'wonder drugs' in the coin of iatrogenic disaster. And she refused to accept the proud dictum of the pharmaceutical public relations man, 'You have to take the risk of side-effects.'

She was not in the least exclusive as regards other therapies if she felt they would benefit a patient. She never claimed that homoeopathy was a panacea, nor was she committed to it as the only form of treatment. She fully recognised that it had limitations, and where these limitations occurred she did not hesitate, because of her basic training, to seek help from other directions. This explains, incidentally, why she was apprehensive about the spread of lay homoeopathy. Although lay homoeopaths do often help their patients, their lack of training in general medicine means that they are unequipped to diagnose with full accuracy. Nor can they discriminate between situations where homoeopathy is appropriate and where it is not.

Throughout Margery's professional life she held to the empirical rather than the theoretical. She knew full well that, in order to convince the unbelieving medical establishment, homoeopathy would have to be 'proved valid' in the language of science. Yet at the same time she agreed with one of her colleagues who said, 'We are trying too desperately hard to justify . . . Let us not forget that we have a therapy that justifies itself by results.'

Some years before her retirement, in one of her addresses, Margery told how she had recently met a consultant who had been a student with her. This lady had been amazed to find that Margery still had the same enthusiasm for medicine as in her student days. 'Everyone else in our year has been disillusioned long ago,' she said. 'Of course they have,' Margery replied.

And why? Because they were sceptical and would not investigate a system that would bring back their enthusiasm, 'a system that can give hope to the most hopeless case and satisfaction and a thrilling life to the prescriber'.

What then was the impetus behind Margery's homoeopathy? How can it be summed up? Lady Namier, for many years her patient, once defined it admirably in the following words: 'Inexhaustible dynamism activated by an insatiable desire to heal. The most complete self-dedication.'

NOTES AND SOURCES

ABBREVIATIONS

BHJ   *British Homoeopathic Journal*

C of H   *The Challenge of Homoeopathy* (Margery C. Blackie, 1981)
originally published as *The Patient, Not the Cure*

CHAPTER 1   *Early Years*

Blackie family history: A genealogical tree of the Compton-Burnett
and Blackie families is included in Vol I of Hilary Spurling's biography of Ivy Compton-Burnett, *Ivy When Young* (1974). This book
also includes valuable information about Dr James Compton Burnett and his family, as well as on the Blackies (pp. 18–44). The 'little
Georgie' incident is from J. Compton Burnett's *Fifty Reasons for being
a Homoeopath* (1934 ed.) pp. 15–18. The descriptions of 'Mr and Mrs
Blackwood' are from *Dolores* (Ivy Compton-Burnett, 1971 ed.) pp.
5–8, 23–29 *passim*. In *Men and Wives* (1931 ed.) 'Sir Godfrey Haslam'
is described on p. 8.

    The Haberdashers' Aske's School: information on Margery's time
there is largely from school records and the school magazine; see also
Marion Spring's *Memories and Gardens* (1964) pp. 24–8 and *Frontis-
piece* (1969) pp. 84–9, also *A short description of the Worshipful Company
of Haberdashers* (H. Prevett, 1971) pp. 24–5.

    Sources of quotations:

'. . . one of those lucky people . . .'/ *BHJ* 1951 p. 174;

'Like should be treated by like.'/*C of H* p. 4

CHAPTER 2   *Medical Student*

The facts of Margery's time as a medical student are taken from her
application for admission to the London (Royal Free Hospital)
School of Medicine for Women, her hospital card, magazines of the

school and annual reports of the Royal Free Hospital. Her first appointment at the London Homoeopathic Hospital (10 April 1924) is recorded in the hospital's 74th Annual Report, p. 15. For background on the status of women in the medical profession see *Elizabeth Garrett Anderson* (L. Garrett Anderson, 1939), *The Life of Sophia Jex-Blake* (M. Todd, 1918), and *Storming the Citadel: The Rise of the Woman Doctor* (E. Moberly Bell, 1953).

Sources of quotations:

'It has often been said . . .'/*C of H* p. 11

'My feet and fingertips . . .'/*Samuel Hahnemann, His Life and Work* (R. Haehl, 1927), Vol I p. 37

'. . . more than two thousand medicines . . .'/*BHJ* 1944 p. 176

'Remember that you will not reach . . .'/magazine of the School of Medicine for Women, November 1921 p. 108

'The first thing women must learn . . .'/L. Garrett Anderson, *op. cit* p. 229

'In my teaching hospital . . .'/*BHJ* 1951 p. 174

'I was interested in homoeopathy . . .'/*BHJ* 1965 p. 222

CHAPTER 3   *Hospital Physician*

The London Homoeopathic Hospital: chronologies of the hospital's history were included in its annual reports in the 1920s. A historical summary is given in the centenary booklet 'The Royal London Homoeopathic Hospital' (1949). Margery described the hospital 'in its heyday' in *BHJ* 1971 (pp. 9–10). For recent developments see *BHJ* 1980 p. 58. Information on the Missionary School of Medicine is from the school's annual reports.

Personalities in homoeopathic history: Dr Frank Bodman's paper 'The Life and Times of Dr Quin' (*BHJ* 1961 pp. 73–82) is the main source of information on homoeopathy in the 19th century and on the royal family's early adherence, also on Dr Quin's career. Dr George Moore (Queen Alexandra's physician) is mentioned in the 75th annual report of the London Homoeopathic Hospital under the heading 'Previous Royal Patronage'. The reference to the 7th Earl of Elgin is based on *Memoirs of 80 Years* (Gordon Hake, 1892), p. 100, and on unpublished correspondence in the Elgin archives. The account of Robert Browning's 'conversion' is from *Elizabeth Barrett Browning: Letters to her Sister, 1846–1859* (ed. L. Huxley, 1929), pp. 289–90. Details of Disraeli's last illness are from *The Life of Benjamin Disraeli* (W. F. Monypenny and G. E. Buckle, 1929) Vol. II, pp. 996, 1052, 1063–4, 1482–3. See also a letter from Dr T. Miller Neatby in *BHJ* 1938 (pp. 232–3).

Physicians at the London Homoeopathic Hospital: appointments are listed in the hospital's annual reports. References to individual doctors in this chapter are as follows: *Dr Clarke*, Margery's memories of him (*C of H* pp. 159–60), his paper 'The Two Paths in Homoeopathy' (*The Annals of the British Homoeopathic Society*, August 1891 pp. 223–35), see also Dr Frank Bodman's Richard Hughes Memorial Lecture (*BHJ* 1970 pp. 179–93); *Dr Wheeler*, obituaries and tributes in *BHJ* 1947 (pp. 1–11); *Dr Borland*, obituaries in *BHJ* 1961 (pp. 133–35 and p. 288); *Dr Bodman*, obituary in *BHJ* 1980 (p. 110) and memorial address in *BHJ* 1980 (pp. 220–22).

Sources of quotations:
'I soon found that it was run . . .'/letter from Dr A. Taylor-Smith in *BHJ* 1961, p. 288
'The spoken word . . .'/*BHJ* 1951 p. 175
'We put up our problems . . .'/*BHJ* 1951 p. 175
'. . . so codified . . .'/Hilary Spurling, *op. cit* p. 98
'ten drug pictures'/*BHJ* 1960 p. 87
'We were quite amazed . . .'/*C of H* p. 163
'Go back and look . . .'/*C of H* p. 162
'No doubt if he had been given *Sulphur* . . .'/*BHJ* 1947 p. 130.

CHAPTER 4   *Into Partnership*

Margery's professional beginnings: for an account of how the Fulham Road practice began see interview in *Newsagent and Bookshop* (4 March 1976, pp. 29, 34). Street addresses in this chapter are taken from contemporary Post Office directories. 'The *Lycopodium* case' is described in *C of H* pp. 110–11 and *BHJ* 1971 p. 6. See also *BHJ* 1951 p. 178. Margery's paper on Asthma was published in *BHJ* 1932 pp. 179–91.

Personalities: for information on Dr G. Campbell Morgan see obituary in *The Times* (18 May 1945) and *Dr Campbell Morgan, A Man of the Word* (J. Morgan, 1951). For details on Sir John Weir see obituaries in *The Times* (19 April 1971) and in *BHJ* 1971 (pp. 103–4). 'The Cure of the Chronic Invalid' was published in *Lyrica Hospitii Homoeopathici* (2nd ed. 1934) pp. 33–8.

Sources of quotations:
Margery's Richard Hughes Memorial Lecture (*BHJ* 1960) is the source of the following:
'. . . because Dr Hughes advised it . . .'/p. 79
'I remember vividly . . .'/p. 81
'. . . a new patient . . .'/p. 87
'those sheets of questions . . .'/p. 87

'She [Dr Banks] kept my feet on the ground'/*BHJ* 1972 p. 67
'I did see a number of cases . . .'/*BHJ* 1951 p. 174
'Since I've started gardening . . .'/*BHJ* 1951 p. 175

CHAPTER 5 *General Practitioner*

For Margery's clinical methods see *C of H*, pp. 57–73. For details of the formation of the Faculty of Homoeopathy see *BHJ* 1944 pp. 2, 3.

Papers by Margery: 'The Clinical Aspect of the Backward Child', *BHJ* 1934 pp. 362–72; 'Rheumatoid Arthritis', *BHJ* 1935 pp. 138–47; 'Helps from the Emanometer', *BHJ* 1941 pp. 210–15.

Personalities: Information on Dr Margaret Tyler is from her obituary by Sir John Weir in *BHJ* 1943, pp. 92–3; for Dr Martyn Lloyd-Jones and his relationship with Dr Campbell Morgan see *D. Martyn Lloyd-Jones: The First Forty Years* (Iain H. Murray 1983), pp. 330–76 *passim.*, see also *The Young Woman who lived in a Shoe* (E. Braund 1984) pp. 23–5.

Sources of quotations:
'It is the mental state . . .'/*C of H* p. 66
'You are appointed . . .'/Report of the 74th annual general meeting of the London Homoeopathic Hospital (1924, p. xii)
'There was the woman . . .'/*BHJ* 1951 p. 10
'if they were given . . .'/*BHJ* 1951 p. 9
'Behind the material world . . .'/BHJ 1939 p. 158
'It will be seen . . .'/*BHJ* 1939 p. 168
'MF Hom.'/*BHJ 1942 p. 167*

CHAPTER 6 *Madame President*

The Faculty officers and Council members during Margery's first year as President are listed in *BHJ* 1949 (p. 310). For her first presidential address see *BHJ* 1950, pp. 15–23. For a full report of the International Homoeopathic Conference in 1950 see *BHJ* 1950, pp. 187–208. For Weir's vote of thanks to Margery see *BHJ* 1950 p. 314.

The Madeira cruise anecdote was often related by Margery, e.g. *BHJ* 1965 p. 222, *BHJ* 1971 pp. 5–6. Background on misconceptions about homoeopathy is from 'The Allopath's reaction to Homoeopathy' (Dr Charles E. Sundell, *BHJ* 1936 pp. 243–51). Margery's account of Hering's proving of *Lachesis* is from *C of H* (p. 38). The Myra Hess anecdote is also from *C of H* (p. 78).

Sources of quotations:
'. . . and now at 98'/*BHJ* 1950 p. 19
'What, after all this . . .'/*BHJ* 1950 p. 23.

CHAPTER 7   *A New Life*

An obituary of Lady Jane Lindsay was published in *The Times* (3 January 1948).

Margery's third presidential address (*BHJ* 1951) is the source of the following:

'If only we could convert an army of young men . . .'/p. 175
'I found her looking and feeling very ill . . .'/p. 177
'Good morning, Mrs Smith, how are you? . . .'/p. 177
'describing homoeopathically is rather like bird-watching . . .'/ p. 178
'The life of the general practitioner . . .'/p. 179

The following are from Margery's valedictory address (*BHJ* 1952):

'. . . what is our object as a faculty . . .'/ p. 69
'We residents looked forward . . .'/p. 69
'Do we have the same effect today . . .'/p. 69
'If I felt . . .'/p. 70

CHAPTER 8   *Classical Homoeopathy*

The visit of H.M. the Queen to the Royal Homoeopathic Hospital was reported in *BHJ* 1956 (p. 47).

Homoeopathy in America: for the Hahnemann bicentenary in the U.S. see *BHJ* 1955 (p. 22). Background on U.S. developments is given in *The Case for Unorthodox Medicine* (Brian Inglis, U.S. ed. 1965). pp. 85–92, also in *Homoeopathy in America: The Rise and Fall of a Medical Heresy* (M. Kaufman, 1971) *passim*.

The British Homoeopathic Journal: Margery mentioned her editorship in a letter to Dr Bodman (7 May 1955), see also *BHJ* 1955 p. 45. For the editorial by her see *BHJ* October 1955, pp. 1–2. Dr Banks's illness is referred to in a letter to Margery from Dr Bodman (3 September 1956).

Anthroposophy: the beliefs, and the deaths, of Primrose and Katharine Compton-Burnett are described by Hilary Spurling in Vol I of her biography of Ivy Compton-Burnett (*op. cit* pp. 252–4); for the adherence of Vera and Juliet Compton-Burnett to anthroposophy see her Vol II, *Secrets of a Woman's Heart* (1984) pp. 54, 290. For information on *Iscador* see '*Iscador* Therapy of Cancer' (Dr A. Leroi, *BHJ* 1965 pp. 27–35), also 'Rudolf Steiner's medical thinking and its relationship to Homoeopathy' (Dr P. B. Engel, *BHJ* 1961 pp. 185–90).

Sources of quotations:
'homoeopathic arrow' and 'orthodox blunderbus'/'Homoeo-

pathy in General Practice' (Dr Hugh L. MacKintosh *BHJ* 1952 p. 153)

'. . . the rapidly enlarging aviary . . .'/*BHJ* 1952 p. 70
'I feel so much better in myself . . .'/*BHJ* 1944, p. 175
'Dr Blackie is the best known . . .'/*BHJ* 1960 p. 141
'We still have those among us . . .'/*BHJ* 1960 p. 80

CHAPTER 9   *Town and Country*

A report by Dr J. E. G. Brieger of the Dress Show at Hedingham, and also of the 'Grand Ball', was published in *BHJ* 1964 (pp. 290–91). The anecdote about Lady Namier is taken from *Iulia de Beausobre: A Russian Christian in the West* (C. Babington Smith 1983, p. 98).

CHAPTER 10   *Royal Physician*

Margery's appointment as Physician to H.M. the Queen was reported in *The Times* on 1 January 1969. The Guildhall reception on 22 October 1970 was reported in *BHJ* 1971, p. 69. H.R.H. Princess Alice's accident in 1965 is described in *The Memoirs of Princess Alice, Duchess of Gloucester* (1983) pp. 187–89. For mentions of the royal family's association with homoeopathy see 'Homoeopathic Medicine, Pharmacy and Lay Organisations: Their Relationship to the Monarchy' (*Homoeopathy*, November–December 1984, pp. 158–59).

The Golden Jubilee Dinner for Sir John Weir was reported in *BHJ* 1960 (pp. 147–55); detailed information on his character is from obituaries in *BHJ* 1971 (pp. 224–28) and *The Times* (19 April 1971). For Margery's obituary of Dr Banks see *BHJ* 1972, p. 67.

Margery's election as Dean of the Faculty of Homoeopathy was reported in *BHJ* 1964 (p. 218), see also an editorial in *BHJ* 1967 (p. 193). The tribute to her talents as a teacher by 'one of the young doctors' was published in *BHJ* 1982 (pp. 69–71).

CHAPTER 11   *Catastrophe*

After the Trident crash the memorial address by Dr L.R. Twentyman was published in *BHJ* 1972 (pp. 130–33), also the poem 'Air Crash' (p. 134). The quotations concerning Dr Kadleigh are from Margery's obituary (*BHJ* 1972 p. 252). The extract from the letter of condolence from H.M. the Queen to Dr Blackie, dated 27 June 1972, is reproduced with Her Majesty's gracious permission. Information on Mr D. W. Everitt is from the obituary by Mr J. B. L. Ainsworth (*BHJ* 1972 pp. 252–54).

The three articles entitled 'The Signature of the Planet Mercury in Plants: capillary dynamic studies', by Agnes Fyfe, were published in *BHJ* 1973 (pp. 201–32) and *BHJ* 1974 (pp. 24–60 and pp. 111–24). With reference to '. . . the outlook seemed dark' see letter from Dr R. A. F. Jack to *BHJ* (1980 pp. 172–73).

For information on the Birmingham symposia and subsequent developments see 'The Resurgence of Homoeopathy in the Midlands' by Dr Jack (*BHJ* 1978, pp. 39–42) also 'At the Growing Edge of Medicine' by Dr R. J. F. H. Pinsent (*BHJ* 1978, pp. 276–78). The letters from Margery to Dr Jack quoted in this chapter were written between 1973 and 1979.

Sources of quotations:

'I am in despair . . .'/Margery to Dr Bodman, 23 March 1974

'We must have basic homoeopathy taught . . .'/Margery to Dr Jack, 17 July 1975.

'No one ever carried out . . .'/Margery's obituary of Dr Askew (*BHJ* 1977 p. 224)

CHAPTER 12 *Apologia*

The original title of Margery's book was *The Patient, Not the Cure*. Reviews were published in *BHJ* 1976 (p. 190); *New Scientist*, 1 April 1976 (pp. 31–2); *Medical News*, 27 May 1976 (p. 12); *British Medical Journal*, 15 May 1976 (p. 1217), see also subsequent letter to *B.M.J.* from Dr C. K. Elliott (3 July 1976 p. 45); *Newsagent and Bookshop*, 4 March 1976 (pp. 29, 34).

The letters exchanged between Margery and Dr Frank Johnson in 1977 were dated as follows: Margery 2 April, Dr Johnson 7 April, Margery 17 April. See also *BHJ* 1950, p. 20, for a statement by Margery: '. . . Does the homoeopath send for the surgeon in a case of acute appendicitis? Yes, immediately.'

Sources of quotations:

'Homoeopathy is not a philosophy . . .'/*C of H* p. 43

'Throughout the history of medicine . . .'/*C of H* p. 2

'. . . 1700 letters'/*BHJ* 1978 p. 165.

CHAPTER 13 *Retirement*

Dr Jack's letter referring to Margery's failing health is dated 30 November 1978. Dr Burger's letter on Margery's resignation as Dean of the Faculty is dated 25 February 1979. For Margery's appointment to the Royal Victorian Order see *Supplement to the London Gazette*, 30 December 1978.

Details of the concert at Snape were given in *The East Anglian Daily Times*, 27 March 1979. The appointment of Margery's successor as Physician to H.M. the Queen, Dr Charles Elliott, was announced in *The London Gazette* on 31 October 1980.

The memorial service for Margery was reported in *The Times* on 26 November 1981. According to Mrs Maddock, the late Bishop Maddock did not know the source of the verse beginning 'My body is the sheath . . .'.

For developments at the London Homoeopathic Hospital see *BHJ* 1980, pp. 118–19; also a report in *The Times* 'Centre for Alternative Medicine' (12 January 1984).

Sources of quotations:

'It is the centre of homoeopathic teaching . . .'/Margery letter to Dr Jack, 3 January 1977

'It was a privilege . . .'/Dr Pinsent's Blackie Memorial Lecture, 1983.

CHAPTER 14   *Achievement*

Sources of quotations:

'In Doctor Blackie's consulting room . . .'/Eric Trimmer in *Medical News* (16 March 1977, p. 15)

'Unless the doctor is utterly devoted . . .'/*BHJ* 1965, p. 220

'You have to take the risk . . .'/article in *The Times*, 'Take the Tablets and the Risk', 1 November 1984 p. 22

'We are trying too desperately hard to justify . . .'/letter from Dr Barry Rose to *BHJ* (1979, pp. 164–65)

' . . . everyone else in our year . . .'/*BHJ* 1965 p. 228

'Inexhaustible dynamism . . .'/letter from Lady Namier to C. Babington Smith dated 5 August 1972.

Index